Yoga

Yoga Nidra & Sutras Patanjali Guide for
Spirituality and Meditation Philosophy

(Holistic Approach To Lose Weight, Heal Your
Body, Revitalize Your Mind)

Mariam Dederer

Published by Rob Miles

Mariam Dederer

Yoga: Yoga Nidra & Sutras Patanjali Guide for Spirituality and Meditation Philosophy (Holistic Approach To Lose Weight, Heal Your Body, Revitalize Your Mind)

ISBN 978-1-989990-61-2

Legal & Disclaimer

The information contained in this book is not designed to replace or take the place of any form of medicine or professional medical advice. The information in this book has been provided for educational and entertainment purposes only.

The information contained in this book has been compiled from sources deemed reliable, and it is accurate to the best of the Author's knowledge; however, the Author cannot guarantee its accuracy and validity and cannot be held liable for any errors or omissions. Changes are periodically made to this book. You must consult your doctor or get professional medical advice before using any of the suggested remedies, techniques, or information in this book.

Table of Contents

INTRODUCTION

There's a lot of hype in the world of wellbeing these days, and you may be puzzled as to where to start in your journey into self-development. Then there's yoga. It really all became popular in the '70s and '80s but the shame of it is the bad reputation that it got, in that people thought that is was the domain of bored housewives or people with too much time on their hands. I remember thinking at the time that it wasn't for me, after turning up for a session and finding that people's descriptions of yoga had been pretty accurate. The class seemed to consist of people trying to better themselves but not in a spiritual way, which is what I had thought yoga should do. These were people dressed in fancy leotards and it was off-putting for me in that I was beginner when they were all intermediate, and my size was what distinguished me from the lithe and lovely middle class housewives trying to find something trendy to do in their spare time.

As the turn of the century arrived, however, people were beginning to see more benefits to yoga than were at first supposed. For example, it was helping people to focus on their lives. It was helping people like me to lose weight and to be less anxious about their lives. The true reason behind yoga practice was beginning to take the world by storm and by the time that I took my first tentative steps into the yoga world, teachers had evolved methods that seemed to be more in keeping with the spiritual side of things. People attending the classes were not there just so that they could say they did something trendy. In fact, those that were looking for that kind of recognition had long since moved onto using the local gym or sports club. Those that were taking part were like me – average people looking for solutions to life's problems and a way forward in stressed environment. Work and home life had evolved and changed. Women no longer stayed home and looked after kids, but were supposed to balance this kind of activity with a full time career and it wasn't easy. Yoga helped considerably to balance the odds, making it possible for participants to become more dynamic than ever before, helping energy levels, spirituality and acceptance of self reach new heights.

As I learned yoga, I also saw that many were actually missing the point of what yoga is all about and for those of you who want to find out what yoga can do for ordinary men and women who have perhaps not taken part in active sports or who have stressed lives, this is probably going to be the book for you. I have written it from the perspective of someone who learned the benefits of yoga and who went on to give classes to those people who were just starting to take lessons and take the yoga seriously as a way to improve their lifestyles. Yoga helps you to lose weight, it helps to balance your thought processes and calms you. It also allows you to feel energized and alive and many of the beginner students who have taken classes with me continue to astound me with the level of yoga they can achieve, once they know what it's all about and realize that yoga isn't sports related. Yes, you will be expected to stretch and bend but it isn't about that. It's about the energy flow through your body and the ability of the mind and body to work in harmony. If you think that's hippy philosophy with no real foundation, think again. It isn't and when you begin to learn yoga, you improve your life and the lives of those around you to such an extent that it will leave you wondering why you didn't take the plunge earlier. I know why I didn't though those times have changed. People who learn today can reap all of the benefits of this ancient practice and that includes you.

If your body has limited flexibility or you find that want to feel fitter and healthier and more in touch with who you really are, yoga incorporates exercises that help you to find that calm within yourself that life on its own isn't allowing you. If you decide to take a class, then this will also motivate you because the people learning today are really seeing the benefits of yoga from many perspectives. For example, ways in which yoga can help you in your life are shown below:

- It can help concentration levels

- It can help in the decision making process

- It can help your health and mental wellbeing

- It can help you to respect your body and keep it in tip top condition

- It can help you to find peace within yourself

Yoga is valuable. Back at the turn of the century when I began my journey into yoga, it started to take the shape that I had originally anticipated from my reading up on the subject although before this time, most people were not ready for that kind of enlightenment and versatility. They are now and that's probably what brought you here, looking for solutions to life's dilemmas and wondering if yoga can help you.

From my experience, I have drawn up a plan which students use in their early days of yoga and which are described in this book. However, you do need to know more about the history of yoga as well and its purpose in order to maximize your experience and know what you are aiming at. This information is also included because it shows you the ways in which yoga came into practice as an aid to spirituality and purpose in life. The movements are easy to follow and the evolution of yoga as a way of life is explained in a way that even the layman can understand.

This book is for you. It's my gift, because yoga has gifted to me its rich heritage and it would be irresponsible to ignore the richness that my experience can add to your understanding and your enjoyment of yoga.

CHAPTER 1: THE MAJOR FEATURES OF YOGA FOR BACK PAIN

Practice of Yoga

My friend Tom provides a dramatic example of the way yoga can speed the healing process. Tom was an eighteen-year-old learning to rock climb when he had an accident that involved a long fall from the top of a cliff. He was lucky to survive; unluckily, he cracked two of his lower vertebrae. Tom's physician happened to be a native of India, and a yoga practitioner. He knew that the boy's injuries could be treated through yoga. At first he taught Tom how to sit properly, so that his spine was properly aligned. This, Tom remembers, was instrumental not only in alleviating his pain but also in facilitating his eventual cure.

The types of prevention

At one time or another almost everyone suffers from back pain, the cause of more lost days of work than anything but the common cold, so the world has turned to secondary prevention as a principal means of addressing it.Yoga is an ideal preventive for those who have either chronic or occasional pain. Tom is an example of someone who learned that yoga can heal, but even now he has to take care of his back and his whole person to prevent old injuries from flaring up. He accomplishes that with yoga.

Secondary prevention involves taking steps to avoid the consequences of a condition. For example, currently there is no cure for diabetes mellitus. But if diabetics carefully regulate their serum glucose and diet, then neuropathy, cardiovascular complications, peripheral vascular disease, and ocular problems can be minimized or avoided.This applies in full force to lower back pain, where reduced activity leads to stiff muscles and joints and to weakness, which are the main causes of chronic back pain.

Overall prevention is impossible. For example, you can't prevent all colds and flu; you can't prevent the accident that causes a broken leg; you can't keep all misfortunes from happening. What you can do, however, is reduce their frequency, severity, and duration. For colds and flu, for example, washing your hands and strengthening your immune system with a healthy diet and lifestyle may make a difference in how often you contract a cold or flu, how badly you suffer, and how long the illness lasts.

Paradoxically, for back pain, prevention constitutes cure. In practicing prevention, your goal is to stop pain from becoming chronic. Yoga does this in eight ways: stretching muscles to reduce spasm and increase flexibility, strengthening muscles and bones, increasing range of motion, sharpening focus, heightening self-awareness, and producing calm. It also improves balance and agility.

You can practice yoga just about anywhere, without spending money, without props, without making noise, and without wearing special garb or giving up your beliefs.

Decreasing Spasm

There are two types of sense organs that record the tension within: One type inside the muscle fibers themselves is called intrafusal fibers. These actually have their own tiny muscles that adjust the tension according to the larger muscle's length. Intrafusal fibers are embedded within the muscles themselves, and when tension increases, either through external pull or because other muscles are contracting, they influence muscles to contract. When there is stress on them, the muscles react by tensing. The intrafusal fibers are dynamic. Tiny muscle fibers inside each intrafusal unit adjust the sensing mechanism to the current conditions of the muscle. Therefore they have a large immediate effect when you move, but that effect gets weaker and weaker as they adjust and as a result movement or tension continues.

The golgi tendon organs, on the other hand, give off a constant inhibitory signal that varies only according to the tension on the muscle. The golgi tendon organs (located in the tendons) cause the muscles to relax when they are stretched. They are static. They produce a constant, unchanging level of signals to the central nervous system to relax the muscle.

At first, the intrafusal fibers actually intensify resistance to stretch, increasing the amount of spasm that is present. But over a short time, their own adjustment mechanism cuts down their input. Usually in less than two minutes the force of the intrafusal fibers falls below the relaxing influence of the golgi tendon organs. Cumulatively, the forces that cause muscles to contract—to get tight when stretched—decrease. The constant inhibitory influence of the golgi tendon organs prevails. The result of this is that stretching a muscle and keeping it in that extended position for any length of time allows relaxation to overtake excitability. The muscle relaxes. Then there is a domino effect that may travel elsewhere in the body, making other muscles become less tense. When you begin a yoga pose, the relaxation that results when the golgi tendon organs go into action is masked at first by the effect of the excitable intrafusal fibers, but that effect falls off quite quickly, while the damping action of the golgi tendon organs continues as long as you are in the pose. Slow and steady wins the day. It is one essential way you can help your body to counter spasm and reduce back pain.

This strategy of staying in a given stretch position for a length of time relies on a reflex, a natural and "hardwired" mechanism that functions at the spinal cord level. It works without our consent. Although we set out to do it on purpose, the effect is mediated on a wholly unconscious level. There is no question that the calm it brings has effects farther up in the central nervous system. We will encounter that benefit of yoga soon enough. But we should first consider another reflex mechanism that can be used to relax involuntarily constricted muscles in spasm.

Every time you flex your elbow, you use your biceps. And every time the biceps contracts and flexes the elbow, its opposite, the triceps, which straightens the elbow when it contracts, must relax and stretch to allow the elbow to bend. Two muscles in this relationship are called "agonist" and "antagonist," depending upon which is doing the contracting. There are many such pairs in the body, of course, and the absence of either partner of the set, through amputation or paralysis, for example, often brings severe spasm to the one that remains.

This opposition is obviously extremely useful. What good is a hand that can grasp if the fingers cannot be opened? These pairs of muscles, mutually dependent for their utility, require precise coordination. Another reflex simplifies the operation: Contraction of one member of the pair works unconsciously to relax the other member of the pair. So as you raise your head by contracting the muscles of the back of the neck, relaxation takes place in the muscles beside the throat that would bring your head down.

Yoga uses this simple but powerful mechanism in many ways. For example, bending forward by contracting the stomach muscles simultaneously relaxes the antagonistic muscles of the lumbar spine. Holding that forward position for a length of time, keeping the abdominal muscles contracted, invokes the relaxing effect of stretching both the golgi tendon organs and the agonist-antagonist mechanism, formidable adversaries of the painful back spasm that we want to vanquish.

The function of Flexibility

A joint in the human body is really miraculous, moving back and forth, as many as hundreds of thousands of times a day for as long as a hundred years, without ever getting stuck! When something does go wrong, however, wear and tear may take place and range of motion may become limited.

Through well-known stretching postures, yoga extends the range of motion of the joints. The inside of the joint capsule, which surrounds the joint much the way a gasket surrounds the juncture between the sink and the faucet, secretes a thick, lubricating substance called synovial fluid, which greases the joint, lubricates it, and allows it to move freely and smoothly. If tendons, ligaments, or muscles associated with the joint become tight, there may not be enough fluid to keep it working properly. Movement may be limited, or there may be pain. No studies have been done on the effect of yoga on synovial fluid, but yoga can safely enlarge the capsule and therefore allow it to continue to function as a secreter and container of synovial fluid.

Ligaments around the joint are made of basically the same material as the capsule, but they are much stronger. Their function is to protect the capsule against overly vigorous movement or movement beyond the normal range of motion. Hatha yoga can stretch ligaments little by little if they become tight or stiff.

Apart from resolving spasm, yoga can also stretch otherwise tense or shortened muscles, changing their length through the continuous pressure exerted on them when an individual attains and holds a particular pose. The stretch itself may engender some discomfort. While that isn't always entirely pleasant, the pain does serve a purpose. It calls attention to the problem area and is likely to provide motivation for an individual to gain control of, say, a particular muscle. Through repeated effort one learns to make that muscle relax. A relaxed muscle can stretch farther. That is key. After controlling the muscle spasm that is so common in back pain, yoga then stretches the muscle farther, so that more movement is possible with less pain. Around joints, yoga increases range of motion; joints at one remove from the painful one adapt by increasing their range of motion to take on some of the strain from the places that are actually producing the pain, allowing them to heal.

Regaining and Increasing the Strength

There are two ways yoga increases strength. First, as with any exercise, muscles get stronger when holding a specific position for any length of time, even for a few seconds, because the body has to fight against the forces of gravity to keep itself in position. In this way, yoga is a little like lifting weights. The counterforce is the weight of your own body and the resistance to movement that different muscles and joints provide. But yoga often increases strength isometrically. Isometric exercise takes place when muscles contract without joints moving. For example, if you lace your fingers together and then try to pull your hands apart, your muscles will contract without any movement taking place. Isometric exercise increases strength with stunning efficiency.

Unlike some activities, the goal of yoga is to gain control, not lose it. Students of yoga who do poses, or asanas, develop personal techniques for relaxing their muscles. These techniques are enhanced by involuntary processes. Nerves have what is called a refractory period. After conducting signals, there is a short period during which they cannot be stimulated to carry any signal, no matter how strong the stimulus. And muscle fibers fatigue from contraction. If one stimulates a previously resting nerve fiber, attached to a calm muscle fiber, it is likely to arouse a maximally powerful contraction. If fifty workmen have the job of moving a heavy block, and some are pulling while others rest from having pulled a moment ago, they will not be as effective as fifty workmen who all pull at once and together. Not only is the muscle stronger; its fibers contract more simultaneously: Strength is more effectively utilized.

Strength is not only a matter of muscles being strong and all their fibers contracting simultaneously; strength is also related to strong bones. The unorthodox and quite sharp pulls that tendons and ligaments make on the bones in the course of doing yoga have been shown in humans and animals to arrest and possibly to reverse osteoporosis.

Everything you need about Calm and comfort in Yoga

It's well known that stress can contribute to back pain and that yoga reduces stress.

Yoga, however, approaches this in a way unfamiliar to Westerners. We believe our minds cause our bodies to move, our brains sending signals down nerve pathways to our muscles. And, of course, that's true. However, in yoga, the opposite also applies. The state induced by yoga in our bodies calms our minds.

Breathing exercises are another resource of yoga that produce calm. These exercises are actually an entire realm of yoga as large as all of hatha, or physical, yoga. Breathing, or Pranayama, is the rhythmical and sophisticated use of one's breath to produce a specific effect. There are centers in the brain that control inhaling and exhaling. Gaining some mastery of these centers seems to control not just breathing itself but a number of other rhythmic and alternating patterns in the brain that, when regulated, produce salutary effects. The individual practicing Pranayama not only becomes calm through breathing in and breathing out regularly; the calm also seems to "spread" through the central nervous system, giving a model of mastery that can be replicated elsewhere in the nervous system. When this is done, it produces an overwhelming level of calm and self-control.

Herbert Benson, MD, of Harvard Medical School described this type of breathing, which is taught in the mantra meditation used in transcendental meditation, in his 1975 book, The Relaxation Response.Basing his thesis on studies at Boston's Beth Israel Hospital and Harvard Medical School, Dr. Benson showed that relaxation techniques such as meditation have immense physical benefits, from lowered blood pressure to a reduction in heart disease, and he made these techniques accessible to everyone. Other introductory texts on Pranayama have been written by B.K.S. Iyengar and Mira Mehta.

Having self-comprehending

There are two more interlocking ways in which yoga helps, especially if you have back pain. A type of self-understanding comes from practicing yoga. Both watching your own reactions to pain and stress and experiencing your own determination to gain mastery over the asanas contribute to your knowledge of yourself. You gain simple understanding of the way your own body works and the things that are better and worse for it, the things that are easier to do and more difficult. This is knowledge in the usual sense of knowing that your back bends only to a certain extent, but it is also knowledge in a deeper sense. You become more than acquainted with yourself; you become familiar. Being familiar with your own body—knowing what you can and cannot do—is a cardinal way to avoid back pain in the first place.

And now for the final advantages to achieving calm. In addition to reducing the drone of anxiety in the background of one's life and increasing the understanding of yourself, yoga contains a means of keeping yourself from getting too excited. Through the practice of yoga you learn how to avoid getting yourself into desperate situations in which you are likely to injure your back or injure it further. Far from trivial, the most important thing in treating back pain (because you can't always avoid it) is to prevent it from becoming chronic. Yoga is the best means I know of for reducing back pain to manageable levels, if not completely abolishing it, and keeping it from becoming a dominant factor in your life.

There are now scientific programs to prove how and how well yoga "works." Yoga actually increases your sense of well-being and self-reliance and is a strong combatant to depression, which may lead to increased somatization of any symptom. But basically it is for aesthetic reasons that people embrace yoga— because of the combination of humility, kindness, consideration, strength, temperance, generosity, and expecting much from yourself and little from others that attracts people to yoga. Essentially people do it not only because they believe they should, but because they want to.

The idea of being able to coordinate one muscle with another presupposes familiarity with one's body, strength and flexibility, focus and self-knowledge. In addition, yoga promotes balance, symmetry, and grace.

CHAPTER 2: STRESS, ANXIETY, AND DEPRESSION RELIEF: EASY YOGA POSES

Yoga is an amazing stress reliever. It eases all anxiety and depression symptoms. It transfers your attention to your breath and body, which reduces anxiety. The yoga poses discussed below curb anxiety, depression, and stress. You can perform them in the order described below, or execute them individually, as you please.

Anjali Mudra

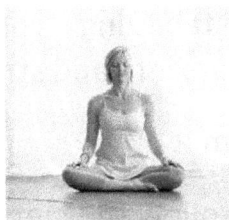

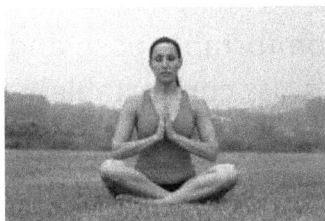

Anjali mudra, also known as salutation seal is a great way to induce a relaxed, meditative state of consciousness and awareness that diverts your focus from all thoughts that trigger stress and anxiety.

Mudra refers to hand positions. In yoga, different nerves in your hands connect to various parts of your brain. By building a connection with those portions, you can produce various desired results.

Anjali mudra is practiced with your hands in front of your heart or heart chakra (a chakra is a point of spiritual power in your body) this helps you establish harmony between the left and right side of your body, thus stabilizing your emotions, which curtails anxiety and stress.

How to Perform It

To practice it, follow the steps below:

1. Sit in a comfortable pose and cross your legs (if this is comfortable). You could open or close your eyes as convenient.

However, for starters, it is best to close your eyes to limit external distractions.

2. Bring your hands to the center of your chestand join them together.

3. Maintain this pose for about ten minutes, and try to relax. Increase your duration by one minute after every two days until you can practice it for 20 to 30 minutes. Performing it regularly will easily reduce stress.

Marjary Asana

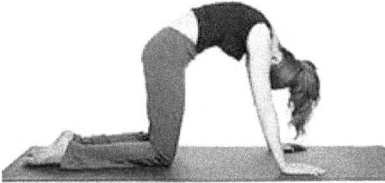

Maryjaryasana, also the cat pose, is a great way to massage your entire body and relax it. It massages your belly organs and spine, and busts away all stress. It also improves your overall health as it stimulates your digestive tract, as well as the spinal fluid.

How to Perform It

1. To perform the cat pose, get on the floor and kneel.

2. Extend your legs backwards and keep your arms straight.

3. Curve your back a little and lower down your head to relax. If you are a beginner, take care when maintaining this pose and place your wrists under your shoulders and your knees right below the hips, so that your alignment is perfect.

4. Maintain this pose for five to fifteen minutes, or for as long as is convenient for you. If you are a beginner, doing it for six minutes in three intervals of two minutes each is sufficient and very effective. As you progress, you can increase its duration.

Uttana Shishosana

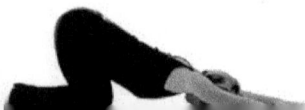

Also known as the extended puppy pose, uttana shishosana is an effective stress relieving pose. It lengthens your spine, calms down your active mind and relaxes your entire body. It eliminates the signs of chronic tension, insomnia, and stress.

How to Perform It

1. To perform the extended puppy pose, kneel on the ground.

2. Open your hips, extend your arms forward, and place them on the floor. Hold this pose for about five to ten minutes.

3. Novices can execute the pose for one minute, take a break, and then do it for a minute more. Start increasing its duration with the passage of time.

Practice these poses every day, or set one pose for one day and do another on the second day and so on. Within two weeks, you will start experiencing amazing results on your stress, anxiousness, and depression.

CHAPTER 3: LOSING WEIGHT WITH YOGA

Another misconception about yoga is that the exercises will not help you lose weight. When you observe a yoga class from afar, you might not see a lot of jumping, running or lifting as you would when you look around a gym, but take a closer look and you will see everyone in class sweating profusely and strongly holding on to a pose.

The body heat you generate through the asanas and breathing exercises do help you burn excess calories. The more intense yoga traditions like Ashtanga and Vinyasa can be considered as cardiovascular exercises because they keep you moving quickly and get your heart rate up. The hot yoga forms are even better for losing weight because you are essentially doing yoga inside a sauna. Bikram yoga is the most popular type of hot yoga there is.

Yoga also relies on body weight and gravity for strengthening and toning, while being a lot safer than using free weights or machines. You might recognize that some of the asanas are the basis for common Pilates exercises and gym forms. A "chaturanga," which you will encounter in Chapter 7, is essentially a variation of the traditional pushup. The Warrior Pose in Chapter 5 relies on a lunge as a base. A burpee is, in essence, a sped up Sun Salutation sequence. Yoga also teaches you proper form and control by making you more mindful of how your body works. This may be quickly glossed over in CrossFit. There is a good reason why your gym trainer emphasizes quality over quantity when it comes to doing reps. The former results in the development of muscle tone and less injury.

The following are other yoga poses that inspired common fitness moves:

The Boat may be familiar to Pilates practitioners as The Hundred. Begin by lying on your mat, then lift your body into a V-shape with your legs and your torso raised at an angle. You are now performing a type of leg lift. Reach your

CHAPTER 4: STRESS, YOUR HEALTH AND YOGA

How Yoga Can Improve Your Overall Health?

If you've been suffering from one or more chronic illnesses, or even if you just don't feel as well as you'd like, I think you'll find this chapter of particular interest. At least, it will give you more reasons to start practicing yoga.

Yoga's beneficial impact on physical and mental health is profound. One of many research examples comes from the National Centre for Biotechnology Information (NCBI). In a 2011 paper from the International Journal of Yoga (IJOY), findings from several dozen studies of the health effects of regular yoga practice were assessed. The conclusions confirmed that health benefits include:

Reduced anxiety and stress

Enhanced mood and increased sense of wellbeing

Alleviated chronic conditions like depression, pain, anxiety and insomnia

Reduced risk factors for heart disease and high blood pressure

Boosted immune system function

Decreased pain and inflammation

Weight loss and a more balanced metabolism

Increased balance and flexibility

Better muscle strength, tone and range of motion, and

Helped access inner strength that allows more effective handling of the fears, frustrations, and challenges of life.

Cautions for Certain Health Conditions

There are precautions and modifications to adapt yoga practice to virtually any medical condition, but it is always wise to be informed, and prepared. Yoga can help.

In the step-by-step pose instructions in the chapters ahead, you will see pose-specific cautions and modifications as much as possible.

Check with your doctor or health care practitioner before embarking on any of the poses included in subsequent chapters to be sure you're getting the best advice.

Osteoporosis, Herniated Disks or Spinal Stenosis

If you suffer from severe osteoporosis or herniated disks, you may wish to avoid forward bends. If you have spinal stenosis, where there is pressure on the spinal chord due to a narrowing in the spinal column, backward bends may cause pain. We use "may" here quite purposefully: there is no conclusive medical evidence that we've found that suggests a direct causal link between these conditions and certain poses. In fact, as many people with these conditions ⬚⬚⬚⬚⬚⬚⬚⬚ from the poses mentioned here as reported pain.

Neck or Back Injuries, Glaucoma or Cerebrovascular Problems

Inversion poses including headstands and shoulder stands have tremendous health benefits, including strengthening the diaphragm, relieving symptoms of bronchitis, emphysema and asthma. For those of you with back or neck problems, glaucoma, or one of the cerebrovascular conditions that affect blood flow to the brain, inversions may not be for you.

Hip Replacements

If you've recently had a hip replacement, use caution or employ a modification in some of the twist poses to be sure you don't damage the prosthetic in your joint.

Multiple Sclerosis

Some physicians recommend that those with MS should avoid Bikram or other

super-focused brain, and heightened sensory awareness that would be put to good use if you were about to be attacked by that tiger.

Parasympathetic

The parasympathetic system, on the other hand, controls the day-to-day functions that are often referred to as the 'rest and digest' state. When your sympathetic system is active more often and for longer periods than your parasympathetic system, your body does not get the time it needs to rest, heal, and regenerate. You become out of balance.

Destructive Coping Mechanisms Versus Yoga

Alcohol, food, drugs, shopping, gambling, eating, even sleeping or exercise, are all used at some time, by some people, as self-medication (or a form thereof) to provide "relief" from the agony of excess stress. These activities are encouraged societally - liquor ads, campaigns to legalize marijuana, the proliferation of fast food outlets, tourist destinations that use gambling as a hook, and so on. There's no end of easy access to the things to stimulate "pleasure" in the hopes of offsetting pain.

I am not judging or begrudging anyone who attempts to combat stress in any of these ways. But these mechanisms are all potentially destructive, causing the body more harm in the long term, compounding the negative health effects of stress and leading to more illness. Exactly the opposite of what was intended.

Self-medication habits are formed and solidify over years, even decades. Making a change in your personal response to stress and the destructive tools you may have been using to cope can be a daunting idea.

So how do you start?

Yoga practice, even one or two times per week, can introduce a sense of freedom, happiness, even euphoria, that immediately brings down stress levels with absolutely no negative side effects. You read that right: freedom, happiness, and euphoria. Who needs anything else after that?

"Yoga has a sly, clever way of short-circuiting the mental patterns that cause anxiety."

- Baxter Bell, MD, Yoga Instructor

Bring Stress Into Balance

It's a mistake to think that the objective is to ▨▨▨▨▨▨▨▨▨ stress. Stress is always present when our lives are full and rewarding. It is about learning how to better respond to stress, which yoga does by teaching your nervous system how to bring itself back into balance. You want your sympathetic and parasympathetic nervous systems to have equal time, not reverse the domination of one over the other.

athletic and reasonably fit. However, there are classes for beginners that you can try to determine if this type will suit you. It is a system of breathing and movement where every movement is incorporated with postures and inhale or exhale. It is traditionally taught using the "Mysore" style where its practitioners are working on their own pace with the guidance of a teacher. It allows beginners to practice together with the advanced practitioners. The Ashtanga yoga has 6-series with set of postures that cannot be interchanged which aim to enhance one's breathing and movement. It also heats the body which purifies the organs, the blood and nervous system.

Bikram Yoga is a modern version of Hatha Yoga that was established during the 1970s. Its classes follow the same format of the traditional Hatha with the same postures and two breathing exercises that last to 90 minutes. Only certified teachers of Bikram can teach this. One of its prominent features is that, it is performed in a heated room same as with the Hot Yoga.

Yengar Yoga is a style that utilizes props in performing asanas. Yogacharya B.K.S. Iyengar developed this style based on Sage Patanjali's yoga principles. The usual props used are wooden blocks, blankets, straps, benches, chairs, sandbags, pillows and bolsters. This style is ideal and safe for beginners and advanced practitioners alike. The props are helping the body to attain a pose's ideal alignment and make the asana easier for students to perform. Likewise, this yoga style is recommended for sick and tired persons at home.

Hot Yoga classes that are generic are not the same with Bikram Yoga although they share numerous features. Unlike the Bikram where a sequence must be strictly followed, the postures in Hot Yoga classes can be changed based on the studio where it is practiced. Usually, its classes are performed in a heated room (105ºF) and with 40% humidity. This is not the type of yoga that everyone enjoys. This is a demanding and very sweaty practice which is not suitable for pregnant women. Among its benefits are mind clarity and balancing the emotions.

Hatha Yoga generally refers to a yoga class that incorporated meditation, Pranyama (breathing techniques) and Asana or postures. It moves at a slow pace which makes it ideal for beginners. The classes vary based on the teacher's approach to Yoga. Moreover, Hatha Yoga is good for injured or unwell persons to help them recover faster.

Kripalu Yoga is a variation of Hatha Yoga which is less physical and gentler. It involves a lot of meditation, breathing work and awakening the body, mind and spiritual awareness. It also promotes emotional well-being and healing. However, this is considered a challenging yoga as it aims to transform the lives of its practitioners.

MASTERING YOGA POSES

To master various yoga poses, you should have the will power, must be physically fit and flexible and have a regular practice. As a beginner, you must understand that your body is unique and has a different ability compared to other people. You can master any pose by being dedicated to practice it.

Practice the pose by holding onto it for at least 10 seconds or depending on your strength. Practice every pose within your body's limits as performing a pose while stretching beyond the body's ability can cause injury. Stretch until you start to feel pain. Repeat the asana based on your body's ability and gradually increase its duration. Most important, do not compare your pace, your body's ability and yourself with other practitioners both beginners and advanced. Let your body adjust to this practice and totally embrace its principles.

Remember that nobody becomes expert on a certain thing overnight. Start today and stop worrying if you can perform Yoga better. You will eventually find an efficient studying texts and scriptures of the yogic tradition. Its approach is the most direct and at the same time, the most difficult. It requires serious study and appeals to people who are intellectually inclined.

TANTRA YOGA- the 6th branch of yoga and the most misunderstand one. It is the ritual's pathways which include the sanctity of sexuality. Among the major branches, this is the most obscure and usually appeals to those who relate with the principles of feminine and enjoys ceremony. Likewise, if you are moved by the importance of rituals and celebrations and find magic in it, this yoga can be the right one for you.

ASHTANGA YOGA- this is the most popular among all the branches of yoga and is widely practiced nowadays. Literally, ashtanga mean 8 limbs. The limbs basically serve as guidelines on the purpose of life and how to meaningfully live it. It also acts as prescription for ethical conduct and moral as well as self-discipline.

Now that you already know the types of yoga and its basic principles, it's time to get ready and prepare for the whole new environment.

CHAPTER 6: HEALTH BENEFITS OF YOGA

Yoga has innumerable benefits to offer. This ancient art has been proven effective for treating various health conditions. It stimulates glands and organs thereby optimizing their function. Regular practice of yoga helps to maintain physical and psychological wellbeing. Keep in mind that Yoga is all about releasing, no need to push or strain, simply relax your body into it and let go with the help of your breathing.

For Overall Health

Yoga oxygenates the body thereby supporting physical and mental health. It boosts blood circulation. It strengthens your respiratory system and greatly reduces risk of respiratory disorders. It stimulates digestive system and promotes optimum performance. It regulates hormone production.

Yoga boosts immunity and prevents illnesses. It supports heart health. It increases spine and joint flexibility. Regular yogic practices tone your muscles and improve muscle strength. It also works great for bone health.

Yoga stimulates your glands and organs and promotes overall health. It improves brain power and focus.

Yoga postpones symptoms of aging. With regular practice, you prevent aging signs such as reduced movement, stiff joints and compromised flexibility. It tones your skin and gives it a healthy glow.

For Health Issues

Yoga aids in weight loss. It also helps to gain weight. In short, it helps to maintain healthy weight. Yoga can help cure insomnia. It can also cure various types of pain including migraine, back pain, neck pain, shoulder pain and leg pain.

Yoga is effective in treating thyroid disorders, eye disorders, menstrual pain

Breathing, meditation, and exercise form the foundation of this practice. Exercises place pressure on glandular systems, increasing the efficiency and overall health of the body. The tradition is passed on from a teacher to a student through oral instruction and physical demonstration. Techniques commonly practiced today are base on collective experiences that developed over thousands of years.

Yoga is a great way to improve your health and wellbeing these days as most yoga positions incorporate many of the practices of the Hindu religion. It has become very popular throughout the world as it is a mind body exercise that benefits the whole body. Yoga is enjoyed by many different cultures of people who do not practice for religious reasons so they have no real understanding of the ancient history or practices of those religions.

Yoga is not just a recent fad, it has been practiced in different cultures for centuries and up to the present, yoga students all over the world are benefiting from it. One reason that Yoga is so popular is that Yoga poses for beginners are very easy to learn, even if you have never taken a Yoga class before.

Another reason for its popularity is that Yoga unifies the mind, body and spirit. Yogis have believed that the mind and the body are bonded into a unified structure. This belief has never failed and changed through the years. The conjugation of your body and your mind is acquired through yoga exercises and techniques.

With the relaxing and unwinding effects of yoga, many health care professionals have been convinced that yoga has also therapeutic results and can be recommended for people with various health problems. Yoga has shown again and again that when performed regularly and properly, an amazing healing power through harmony is attained. So if you experience health issues over a long period of time, you may want to start practicing yoga poses for beginners and apply the healing powers of Yoga to yourself.

When people first hear of yoga, they wonder how Yoga exercises are done and which poses are best to start with. So lets give you some insights. If you want to practice yoga for beginners, you must trust that yoga is effective and will help you to be cured or be empowered.

Those of you that are not familiar with the Yoga poses for beginners now have the right mind set. But there is more to consider.

It has been proven that the yoga poses are extremely useful when it comes to maintaining a high level of joint flexibility. Although yoga poses for beginners are basic exercises that can be done by everybody, done right and regularly Yoga can slowly contribute to a healthier lifestyle, and its positive effects will multiply when Yoga is exercised over and over again.

Yoga poses can be very stimulating and exciting to learn. Good news is that beginners will never find it hard to keep up with Yoga exercises because basic positions are easy to learn. If you are ready to learn yoga poses for beginners, you can do so easily at home or by visiting an exercise group where yoga is taught by a professional trainer.

Some basic yoga positions include standing and seated poses, forward and backward bends, balance and twisting. These yoga poses are not that far from the positions used by more advanced yoga practitioners. Yoga exercises range from simple to extreme poses and positions, that are handled in the advanced training.

Another questions many Yoga beginners ask is: how long should I practice the exercises? The rule of thumb is not to drain your body. Also, beginner's should give their body some rest between the exercises.

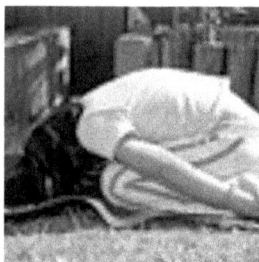

This kind of exhausting schedule is repeated day after day with little time designated for rest and relaxation.

While this goal-oriented life provides rewards, there are side effects. Many of these children with hectic schedules suffer from anxiety, depression, eating disorders and weight issues.

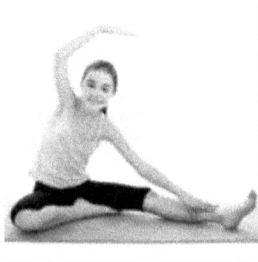

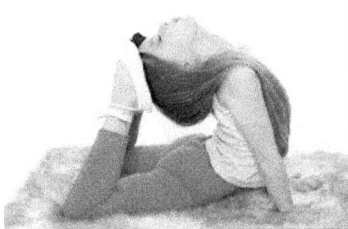

Indeed, the childhood years are an intense duration of emotional, social, and intellectual growth. Often when children are faced with stress their bodies' sympathetic nervous system is triggered.

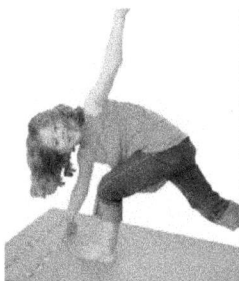

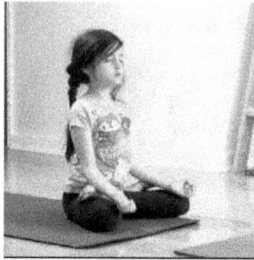

This can result in an increased heartbeat and raised blood pressure which, over time, plays a role in the immune system functioning, disease fighting capacity, self-esteem, and mental and emotional health.

Research indicates that the increasing demands placed upon children in the school system have adversely affected students' behavior, self-esteem, concentration, educational success and psychological balance.

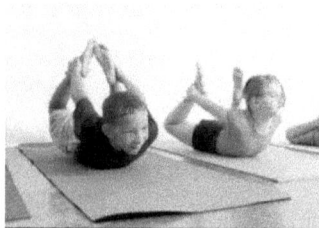

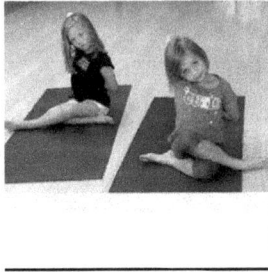

Among children who practice yoga, there is believed to be a reduction in anxiety, stress, behavioral issues, emotional issues, and even bullying and violence.

In this day and age, children who suffer from these issues are often placed on medication. Yoga is an all natural, comprehensive way to address a myriad of problems today's children face. It allows them to slow down and focus on themselves as a person instead of a product of society.

Intense and demanding schedules can easily contribute to childhood obesity. The more children are inundated with the pressure to achieve, the less time they may have to devote to physical exercise.

They may also try to soothe themselves or self-medicate with food that is comforting but not healthy. In what downtime they do have, they are likely to devote it to playing video games, watching television or surfing the net.

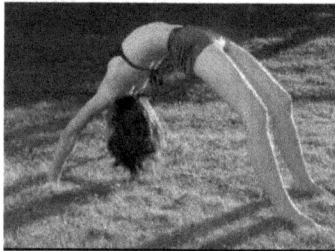

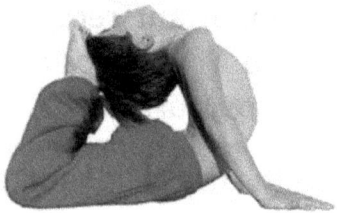

Research shows that an overwhelming number of children ages 6-19 are either overweight or obese. Most of these children do not fulfill the lowest recommendations for normal physical activity (one hour daily) established by the Academy of Pediatric Medicine.

Coupled with a lack of exercise, poor eating habits are a major contributor to childhood obesity. Buyers today are inundated with marketing and advertising that promotes overly processed and refined food as well as convenience food that is aimed to fit into our busy lifestyle.

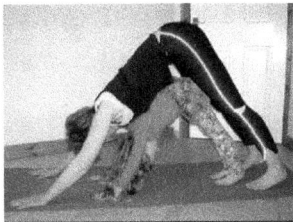

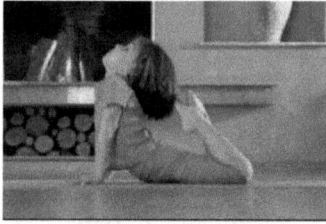

While yoga is often perceived as a passive exercise, in reality it is very active. The fact that is addresses the entire body; mind and spirit indicate that it may have the most significant effect on childhood obesity.

Yoga helps to regulate the appetite in children. It encourages them to make healthier choices and begin to understand how certain foods make them feel when they eat it. Yoga has also been known to completely change one's food desires. A child, who once craved salty, greasy, or sugary food, may begin to crave fruits and vegetables.

Hence, actively participating in yoga on a regular basis is one way to encourage youth to work in the direction of the suggested one hour of physical exercise daily.

It offers children an alternative to a rapid change of lifestyle. Rather than having them completely stop eating junk food, reduce their portions and begin running and other types of intense exercise, yoga takes a more organic approach by allowing the yoga to help children make the decision to be healthy on their own, both consciously and subconsciously.

Yoga and the Body Acceptance

One more part of yoga that's very therapeutic for youngsters is the practice of awareness, or even Meditation. Via this training students start to get in touch with and listen to their inner thoughts.

Yoga fosters tolerance and empathy. It boosts children's awareness which aids in self-compassion as well as concern with others.

Benefits for Children

progression geared toward interpersonal and social skills. It helps boost a child's self-confidence resulting in less awkward interactions with peers and adults.

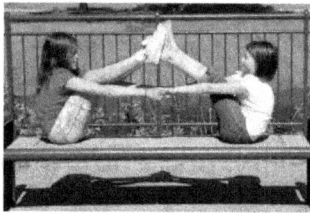

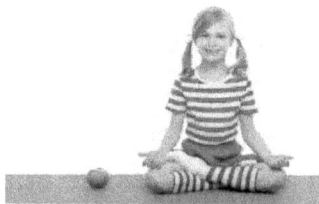

Individuals having learning difficulties or even behavior challenges are known to have benefitted from yoga.

Research indicates that students with attention deficit disorder and attention deficit hyperactivity disorder who practice yoga report a reduction in their symptoms and an increase in their ability to focus, pay attention and be productive.

In addition, yoga has been utilized to assist at-risk youth around the U.S. has been proven to assist students who struggle in the traditional school setting.

The Reason Yoga Really Works

Yoga functions by fostering and interaction between the whole mind and body, supplying energy for all types of personalities and learning styles. It caters to the visual, kinesthetic, audio, and natural components in a child.

By encouraging children to call upon their individual inner resources—
such as soothing mechanisms, focus, and as self-acceptance—yoga enables them to really gain a sense of their place in the world and among society.

How Yoga Works

When teaching yoga to children, it is essential that you have a safe and accepting environment. Directing courses which can be focused on children of all personalities, fitness levels and experience encourages a confident interpersonal atmosphere.

Thankfully, yoga does not have to be limited to a standard setting like a studio or a gym. Since there is little to no equipment necessary, yoga is perfectly suitable for a regular classroom or outdoor space.

As with any type of exercise, adaptations may be required depending on the needs of students. These might include not going as deep into a pose in the beginning or holding a posture for a shorter amount of time then gradually increasing the depth and length of time.

Yoga when practiced by children makes use of ⬚⬚⬚⬚⬚⬚⬚(postures), focused on specific parts of the body, and ⬚⬚⬚⬚⬚⬚⬚⬚⬚(inhaling and exhaling methods) in order to encourage them to help combine their bodies with their minds and their spirits.

The Body

Yoga ⬛⬛⬛⬛ those that involve standing and sitting or lying down, first help to address problem in your physical body. Just as there are many types of yoga, there are thousands of yoga postures.

By practicing and even mastering physical postures, you can learn to control your mind. For example, learning to be still in a posture by ignoring mild discomfort or not wiping sweat away from you face, can translate into your life outside of yoga by teaching you to ignore insignificant distractions and annoyances.

The Mind

In turn, yoga focuses your mind by requiring you to concentrate on particular parts of the body. For instance, you may be directed by the instructor to focus intently on your back or sink deeply into the floor.

This focus helps to keep mind sharp. There is no attention given to outside

face and body. In other instances, the period of ⬜⬜⬜⬜⬜⬜ will either be accompanied only by soft music or be in complete silence.

The idea is to let any thoughts you may be having simply appear and then vanish. This is helpful in moving you into a complete calm relaxation and soothing condition so you can carry that peace with you when you leave. ⬜⬜⬜⬜⬜s generally the final part of the yoga practice.

The Spirit

Yoga utilizes controlled and conscious breathing as a way to combine your mind, body, and spirit. The particular breathing strategies are called ⬜⬜⬜⬜⬜⬜⬜; prana signifies energy or life force.

Ancient Hindu wisdom asserts that by controlling your breathing you control the vital circulation of energy throughout your body.

It is that conscious breathing that we practice that helps us to focus on muscles which are working during our ▯▯▯▯▯▯▯ and during ▯▯▯▯▯▯▯▯ when we attempt to decrease our heart rate, calm our mind, and create a deep, internal peace and relaxation.

Cautions for Yoga Exercises

Although most forms of yoga are safe for anyone to practice, a few are usually strenuous and could not be right for every person.

Specifically, elderly patients or perhaps those with range of motion issues might want to consult with a health professional before choosing yoga being a treatment option.

Those who suffer from back injuries or sciatica pain may need to avoid certain postures. For sufferers of mild to moderate pain, stiffness and bodily stress, yoga can be a miracle worker.

Yoga has been known to help practitioners cope   with depressive disorders, anxiety, and stress. While it may not completely eliminate these issues, although it is possible, it certainly can help to manage them

More and more studies point to mental and physical wellness as not only being closely allied, but essential for optimal wellness.

When you look at all the ways that yoga can   increase your   well-being,   you probably notice a lot of overlapping. The physical, mental and spiritual benefits are intensely interwoven.

This   is one   of   the   fundamental understandings   of   yoga--Everything is connected—the bottoms of your feet to the top of your head, the state of your physical well-being to your sense of peace and happiness, your peace and happiness to that of your community and your world.

This kind of synergism is the most significant aspect of a healthy yoga practice. The physical, mental and spiritual healing that takes place is unique to the practice. You will learn to heal yourself from the inside out.

even help you keep most of that flexibility even as you age.

☐Strength. Many of the yoga poses that you'll be doing require strength to support the weight of your body in different ways. There's balancing on one leg or supporting your entire weight with your arms. At first, it might be a little tricky to master, especially if you have never been the type to do any exercise. However, with repetition, you will be able to build up your strength slowly and the change will be very noticeable. You will strain less and might even begin looking for more challenging poses to do.

☐Muscle tone. A byproduct of your own strength building. Since you will be using your muscles more, this also helps in toning them. Arms, legs, the buttocks area - all of these would benefit from constant yoga practice. You can expect them to become leaner, longer and shapelier.

☐Balance. Think you're clumsy? Always tripping? Has it gotten worse the more you got older? Well, don't fret! Balance is something that you can always remedy and improve. Some people practice sports for this reason. However, for those who prefer something quieter and calmer, yoga has the answer. The poses can help you find your balance, giving you more confidence with each step. As you progress, you will also learn more about core strength and this can boost your balance even more.

☐ Joint Health. People who have arthritis will certainly benefit from regular yet gentle yoga practice. It would help improve their mobility and even help decrease some of the pain associated with the issue. Yoga's breathing exercises can help put them in a calmer state of mind; less frustrated about their situation and help free them of any mental issues that they might be experiencing because of arthritis symptoms. People who have carpal tunnel syndrome will certainly benefit from yoga as well.

☐Pain prevention. With the increase in both your flexibility as well as strength, this can also help with preventing different kinds of back pain. This often happens to people who spend a lot of time sitting, whether they do it while working on the computer or driving. Spinal compression and tightness can happen and cause pain but you can prevent it with yoga. Aside from that, yoga can help improve your alignment and keep your spine healthy.

☐Better breathing. Breathing should be easy, as anyone would say but a lot of us actually do not give much thought to how we are doing it. Yoga breathing exercises such as pranayama bring the focus on developing a healthier, more beneficial way of breathing. This affects the entire body and helps calm the central nervous system whenever we feel tense or anxious. If you are experiencing some allergies, certain types of breathing can also help clear nasal passageways. Needless to say, the simple act of breathing, when yoga is applied, can have both mental and physical benefits.

Mental Benefits:

☐Mental calmness. The yoga practice of asana can be very physical. In doing so, you're concentrating heavily on what your body is doing at the very moment and the act alone can bring calmness to a weary mind. Yoga can also provide you with a number of different meditation techniques. Watching your breath and disengaging from thoughts that no longer serve you are just two of the things you will eventually learn. These skills will prove to be useful in many different ways. For calming an anxiety attack, helping with insomnia and even dealing with both physical and emotional pain.

☐Body awareness. Costant practice of yoga can help you develop an increased body awareness. The small aches and pains, anything that might feel off. Overtime, it will also help increase your comfort level in your own body. You will

provide you with. In the following chapters, we will focus more on two in particular: weight loss and stress relief.

CHAPTER 10: A FEW BASIC RULES

Thousands of yoga students all over the world have gained tremendous benefits from these techniques and many have learned even the difficult postures with ease. The way you practice a particular posture is not as important in determining results as is repetition of the daily routine. The exercises must be done regularly.

Remember that the exercises and the deep rhythmic breathing should be practiced together; the additional supply of oxygen thus brought into your system will cause your glands, muscles, and nerves to function more effectively.

A daily routine of the various postures, correct breathing plus a proper diet will maintain your body's proper weight and shape. A stout person will lose weight whereas a thin person will gain missing pounds. Your posture will improve, too. These postures or asanas will give you a physical inner balance that will help you to relax, concentrate, and meditate.

1. If you have any health problems, be sure to consult your doctor before you begin to exercise.

2. Exercises should be done on an empty stomach, the first thing upon arising or before retiring; in any case before the three principal meals.

3. Do the exercises in a well-ventilated room, or outdoors if the weather permits.

4. Wear comfortable clothes.

5. Choose a surface that is not too hard or too soft. Use a blanket or a mat to do the exercises on.

6. Rest in between the various postures so that you don't get tired. These postures

are designed to give you a feeling of comfort and relaxation, not fatigue. Every posture should be combined with deep rhythmic breathing.

7. Most of the breathing exercises are done in a standing position; however, they can be done sitting in a chair, keeping your spine straight, or lying in bed flat on your back.

8. The postures are done lying or sitting on the floor in some instances; in other instances, standing. However, they can also be done sitting in a chair or lying in a couch or a bed if you have difficulties in the beginning getting to the floor. A slant board is useful for those having trouble getting to the floor. Lie with the head down, relax and do breathing exercises on it daily.

9. Until you reach perfection, it is impossible to practice all the postures at one time; do the ones that are easy for you. Then, after you have made progress, include the others.

10. No matter how little time you can devote in the morning to practice, never neglect to do the breathing exercises upon arising and finish with the vocal exercises.

11. From 15 to 30 minutes is sufficient for an average session. If you don't have that much time, even five minutes a day will prove beneficial. But never miss a day.

12. Do not exercise more than a total of one hour a day.

13. Proper food and rest and enough sleep are of paramount importance for the program to work effectively. The average person requires about eight hours of sleep each night. Sleep before midnight is considered the best.

14. Relax the body before you begin to exercise.

CHAPTER 11: WHY SHOULD YOU PRACTICE YIN YOGA

Yin Yoga has multiple benefits – physical, mental, emotional and spiritual. While there is more demand for the physical, emotional, and mental benefits, it is the spiritual benefits that bring you far-fetched goodness. When we start to discover ourselves through the spiritual aspects, we learn to live in this moment. When we learn to become mindful, life becomes a smooth, happy flow!

Yin Yoga is for anyone and everyone out there. We can do it when we are hyperactive or extremely fatigued. We can do it to calm your excess energy or to satiate our energy cravings. Since this style of Yin Yoga works on our connective tissues, the poses are held for at least 5 minutes. This longer period will give enough time for the tissues to warm up and respond in a slow and steady way.

Our body will express its gratitude by lengthening and strengthening itself, which is the physical benefit all of us expect. Just remember that all you have to here is to let go of your ego and surrender yourself to the pose, allowing the stress to build up in an easy way, thereby making the body supple and flexible.

Let's take a closer look at some of the benefits you can reap through regular Yin Yoga practice:

Physical Benefits

Physical benefits are more tangible, and hence we tend to crave for those.

Yin Yoga:

☐ Removes deep blockages in the connective tissues to encourage the energy flow

☐Increases circulation

☐Improves flexibility

☐Facilitates myofascial release

☐Improves body posture

☐Increases suppleness and strength

☐Gifts greater joint mobility

☐Stimulates better digestion

☐Promotes detoxification

☐Lessens inflammation

☐Enhances immune system

☐Improves blood pressure

☐Lowers heart rate

☐Brings balance to the internal organs

☐ Encourages unobstructed flow of prana or life force through meridian stimulation

As the poses involve breathing, it improves your lungs and respiratory health.

Mental & Emotional Benefits

These are not as tangible as physical changes, but yes, a calmer, less stressed mind is sure to boost the physical benefits!

Yin Yoga

☐Encourages to create a safe space in the mind

☐ Teaches to observe the emotions as they are

☐ Encourages to let go of unwanted emotions and feelings through conscious surrendering

☐Increases tolerance and patience

☐Eases stress, anxiety, and restlessness

☐Harnesses the monkey mind

☐Improves focus and concentration

☐ Helps to develop emotional maturity and resiliency

☐Boosts confidence

Spiritual Benefits

The most important benefits Yin Yoga gifts are enhanced self-consciousness and an increased mindfulness. Mindfulness is nothing, but just living this moment without trying to analyze and judge it. This yoga form is a kind of active moving meditation. Studies suggest that regular meditation could activate the brain, stimulating the release of various neurotransmitter enzymes that enhances mindful awareness.

So, in short, Yin Yoga

☐Helps to stay grounded

☐Helps to become more mindful

☐Enhances self-compassion

☐Releases ego

☐ Coaxes to let go of criticisms and judgments

☐Encourages to accept things and people 'as is'

☐ Teaches to acknowledge, accept, and nourish ourselves

☐Encourages gentleness and kindness

☐Opens the heart

☐Helps you know yourself

The best part of Yin Yoga is discovering ourselves and accepting us as we are. And, to experience this benefit, we have to know certain things about practicing this yoga form. While there are no hard and fast rules to the practice, these factors could act as guidelines to help us enjoy better practice.

CHAPTER 12: CLEARING YOUR MIND

By practicing yoga, your mind will become clearer. The concept of yoga and its moves encourages you to focus on your body and breathing. With this concentration, other thoughts and worries are swept aside and your focus is on what you're doing in the moment. By clearing your mind, you will feel more calm and relaxed, helping you to rest better and have peace of mind in a busy world.

As with the past chapters, I'm going to focus on a few yoga poses that will be helpful when it comes to clearing your mind. These are poses that you might want to try when you need to relax before doing other yoga exercise or in the spur of the moment when everything seem overwhelming. By clearing your mind, you will be on your way to living a more peaceful, less stressful life.

The Tree Pose

The tree pose is a one-legged pose. Just by concentrating on keeping your balance on one foot should help you clear your mind of anything else. With this pose, take your right foot and place it on the inner thigh of your left leg. Put your arms above your head and hold this pose while breathing in and out. Try holding this pose for as long as possible. Switch legs if necessary.

The Eagle Pose

The eagle pose starts out by using the chair pose. Once in the chair pose, wrap your right leg around your left. Wrap your right arm around your left arm, trying to bring your palms together. Dip down and hold the pose as long as possible, taking slow breaths.

The Warrior II Pose

Take a step back from standing position so that your back leg is parallel to your front leg. Bend your front knee at a ninety degree angle. Spread your arms so that one is reaching forward and one is reaching backwards. Hold this pose while concentrating on your breathing. Switch legs so that you're in the opposite position.

Doing yoga to clear your mind combines basic moves with breathing to help calm and sooth you. It makes you feel like you're in control and will help you to do away with the stresses of the day. Consider doing yoga to clear your mind before you engage in the other forms of yoga. It will help your concentration and help you meditate and become more rested, making the workout much more enjoyable.

CHAPTER 13: TIPS FOR HATHA YOGA

Hatha yoga refers to any type of yoga that makes use of asanas (postures). If you want to see the benefits of Hatha yoga then it is important to practice regularly; you should be aiming for at least three sessions of 30 minutes a week, although a session once per day is even better.

Moreover it is best to consuming any food or drink for at least 1 hour before practicing. Some of the postures in Hatha yoga can be very uncomfortable with a full stomach and your flexibility will be hampered. Ideally it is best to wait for even longer than one hour, but you might have to compromise depending on your schedule. Owing to this, many people choose to try practice yoga as the first activity of their day, whilst their stomach is empty.

Many yogis also advocate a vegetarian diet, due to the belief that it is gentler on

107

the digestive system and stomach and therefore promotes overall bodily health.

Whilst you want to challenge yourself during yoga, it is also important not to push yourself too far. Deep stretching can be uncomfortable, but it shouldn't be painful. Pain is a signal that something is amiss and you shouldn't ignore it. It may be the case that your form is poor and you are applying pressure to joints and ligaments in the wrong places. Alternatively, areas of your body may be weak or damaged to begin with. Regardless, apply a little caution and common sense when dealing with pain.

Whenever you practice Hatha yoga, you will need a yoga mat. The yoga mat is particularly important for protecting the knees, back and ankles from being bruised or damaged when you rest your weight on them against the floor. The yoga mat also helps improves friction and makes it easier to maintain certain postures, whilst softening the impact if you fall or break a pose suddenly.

If a posture is too difficult for you, then there are usually numerous alternatives that are less strenuous, but work on the same regions and areas of the body. Owing to this, don't worry about it. If you find yourself struggling too much, consult a yoga teacher or attend a yoga class to get professional advice.

On top of this, please be aware that yoga is for both sexes. To a certain extent, Western society perceives yoga as a feminine activity, for hip spiritual women. Yet the original yogis were almost all men and many of the most practiced and certified yogis are also male. Yoga should not be categorized with one gender or another and you should be able to find classes which tailor for both sexes, or men and women in separate groups.

Although Hatha yoga's primary focus in on the body, it is wise to meditate or calm yourself before entering a Hatha yoga session. All Hatha yoga should be undertaken mindfully, with a gentle awareness of the movement and

Finally, as a parting note, you need to practice your Hatha yoga in good faith. It's easy to be doubtful about yoga if it is your first time practicing and this can affect your success. At least to begin with, abandon your skepticism and you will find yoga a more rewarding and spiritual experience.

CHAPTER 14: FOOD AND YOGA

Diet and food play a crucial role in yoga. The impacts of poor nutrition and inappropriate nutrition uncover themselves in unpleasant appearance and in flawed behavior and thinking. According to the principles of yoga, food is categorized as Rajasic, Tamasic and Sattvic, which is the ancient adaptation of the Good, the Bad and the Ugly.

Sattvic Yoga Foods

These are food items which are prepared fresh with limited seasonings or spices. These foods maintain their nutritional value since they are cooked very simply. One of the most delicious and nutritious foods with great benefit on the overall body health is Sprout. The principles of yoga highly recommend Sattvic foods.

Rajasic Yoga Foods

These food items are also commonly referred to as foods for kings or of individuals who have energetic or restless dispositions. A huge selection of foods cooked through various methods – fried, baked or highly seasoned, form this yoga food category. Also under this category are processed beverages, alcohol and sweets. By and large, these food items causes additional weight and fats to the body. These foods lead to a feeling of uneasiness after eating and thus produce a lethargic disposition.

Tamasic Yoga Foods

This category includes non-vegetarian and vegetarian foods which are cooked with hot seasonings, salts and excess spices. As a general perception, these types of foods cause a feeling of laziness to those who eat them. Foods under this category lead to intolerant and rough temperament.

Yoga Diet – Foods to Stay Away From

Poor quality oils, margarine and animal fats

White flour and white sugar

Over-spiced foods

Old, stale and over-reheated foods

Genetically engineered foods

Irradiated and microwaved foods

Eggs, fish and meat

Fried foods

Factory farm dairy products

Canned foods (excepts naturally canned tomatoes, vegetables and fruits)

Processed, artificial foods

Artificial sweeteners

Coffee, tea, tobacco, alcohol and all stimulants

Yoga Diet – Foods to Eat

and balance is the key. This should not only apply to the amount of food but also on the seasonings and other flavorings that are found in it. Excess grease, heavy spices or an overload of spices are not part of a yoga diet, but only fresh pure food items for their nourishment. Overloading your taste buds or your plate places a danger on your mind and disposition.

When Should You Eat

Yoga experts strongly suggest that you must not eat foods 2 to 3 hours prior to a yoga class. Some yogis further recommend that you eat food items that are easy on the digestive system and your stomach. Suggestions include foods like toasted whole-wheat bread, hummus, veggies, rice, low-fat yogurt, apples, pears, oatmeal and bananas. Pre-workout snacks must include foods with low glycemic index and you must avoid simple carbs and sugars such as white bread, sweets and donuts.

Rule Exceptions

Because of health issues, food allergies as well as other factors, a strict yoga diet will not be beneficial for everybody. This is but alright as there are yoga diet variations where yogis can consume meat or fish in order to stay focused and healthy. What's important is that you listen to your body and customize the diet according to your body's needs, rather than sticking to a diet regimen which will only make you feel sick, weary or weak.

CHAPTER 15: YOGA POSES TO PRACTICE

Yoga continues to be around for thousands of decades, and how it may be seen as a tendency until now is indeed remarkable! It was able to continue developing at this constant speed since it has been applied for such a prolonged period of time. For that reality, the commonly used varieties of Yoga as of late which frequently requires stretch jeans, comfortable mats and plenty of movements - are almost new.

These innovations do not have a tendency to vitiate the original real centers (asanas) of Yoga. Indeed, robust, flexible systems will be, for that very least developed by physical yoga, best results still benefit from the yoga practice that is a lot more than mental. Yoga routines must require religious enlightenment at some time and a peaceful, open-mind. However, in the beginning of yoga practice, whatever reason one may put up is not unreasonable. And with the basic, this training also needs to start like several other activities. Novices should start with these 5 standard poses and so, yoga poses.

Wide Leg Forward Fold or Prasarita Padottanasana

To newcomers with hamstrings, this type can provide just a little stress in the beginning. This present can be carried out in different versions, but don't believe that this should require hands or head-on -the ground forms straight away.

Getting into the correct form:

With legs wide open, stand with your hips on your mat. The neck should be together along with your back. Legs should be maintained parallel at all times.

With your eyes shut, try and picture the feet like a tripod - with the last one-under your little foot, another level at the mat under your toe and also one pointed at your heel. Root all of these three things on to the bottom.

Breathe deeply and see that you're pulling the roots from the level you have established under your feet unto your sides. This may likely trigger the muscles in your feet and allow you to create a good alignment.

Exhale, while maintaining your back immediately, fold the body forward at your sides.

If you're able to manage, provide your hands all the way to the floor. Try this when you are currently maintaining your extended spine.

If you're unable to reach the surface, fold your legs with your palms placed on your legs.

A few ambitions should be realized while you are retaining this offer.

Your spine prolonged at all times or has to be stored prolonged - this promotes greater back alignment and strength which could help prevent back injury.

The tripods rooted on the floor must be managed. The strength presented in this particular kind must market result from these points - this promotes legs energy, better leg stance that can avoid incidents and keeps you effective within the pose.

Breathe.

Crescent pose

Crescent offer will be the most preferred starting form in most yoga classes. Before engaging in other more complex forms for flows both utilized or poses. A forward position lunge with hands extended expense could be the basic kind of the crescent present.

Having the proper form:

From a forward bend, move your right knee backward, folding into your left calf for a few minutes.

Take your time in stabilizing your lunge. Make certain that both of the feet are firmly planted, your legs are solid and your back extended.

You can release your back knee to the floor if chosen. While lifting up, your system breathes and place your hand on your front knee.

Within the next breath, try increasing your hands overhead, straight up out of your shoulder with palm facing in, if the configuration seems great.

To put to an end, lift your heart up then draw down your neck on your own back. Decrease the back of your leg for the soil when you consider the initial step of your leg back for the lunge, if the position lunge is somehow difficult.

Remember:

A strong base could be the key to being a powerful soldier. Keep these toes deeply grounded to the terrain while drawing strength up to your hips. This can help you align your presence correctly to give security while you're involved with it.

Back shoulder must be ripped down and back. There may be a tendency of your shoulder rolling forward, let it.

Expand your arms entirely from your fingertips. Soldiers don't have arms that flop.

The look you have to agree to is an important element of the present, and never an easy one. It may not be easy for us to retain our eyes staring fixedly at a single spot without getting it distracted rather than allowing it to walk around. You'll need the concentration that a soldier needs to have if it is seeking at its victim, breathing in that same spot.

Child's Balasana or Cause

A child's pose is another kind of yoga pose for novices. This can be a cycle where you can manage to have a remainder or even the period to cool off. Throughout a yoga school, you will be motivated to take if you ever chose to take a break, this offer. This works like a break pose in class, part of the program or whether necessary.

Stepping into it:

Perform a kneeling position, then fold forward. Achieve your arms out until your temple in front of you can touch the bottom.

If you learn it difficult to kneel down, it is possible to place a stop or a rolled up where you prefer or quilt above your calves, or perhaps a blanket underneath your hips.

Both hands could serve as being a stop support if planting your forward to the mat is annoying.

Relax your entire body and then give attention to your breath. This type isn't a working pose; it is a relaxing pose. So, should you ever feel exasperated, you have to regulate the offer.

Yoga could be tough at first but with little endurance around the range, everything works out because you can want it to be!

CHAPTER 16: THE ASANAS

The asanas are now being practiced worldwide and have been adapted in the physical fitness industry. You must understand that this is only one of the eight limbs of yoga. Asanas or physical postures are important in executing the other styles of yoga. Asanas are defined by types, benefits, anatomy, and many more.

Poses by Type

There are many kinds of asanas and they depend on your initial pose upon doing the exercise and what you aim to achieve. These poses include standing, arm balance, balancing poses, binding, chest opening, core yoga poses, forward bend, hip opening, inversion, pranayama, restorative, seated, strengthening, twist, backbends and bandha.

Samples of Standing Yoga Poses

1. Mountain Pose (Tadasana)

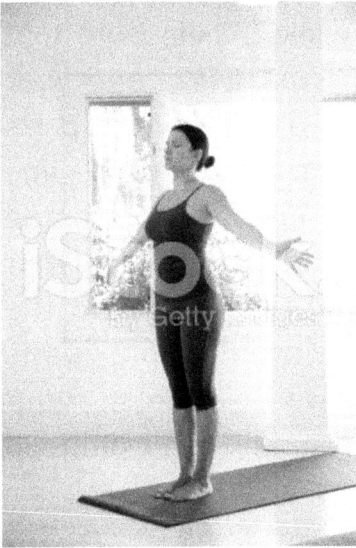

Stand straight with the bases of your big toes touching and the second toes are parallel to each other. Lift and spread your toes and move the balls of your feet and slowly, put them back again to the floor. Begin rocking your weight by moving your feet to the front and back and then from side to side. Gradually reduce the frequency of the swaying of your body until you are standing still and your feet are carrying your weight in a balanced manner.

Lift your kneecaps, while making sure that your thigh muscles remain firm and your lower belly is relaxed. Lift the inner parts of your ankles. Envision that there is a line of energy from your inner thighs to the groins, going through the core of your torso, to the neck, all the way up to the crown of your head. Move the upper parts of your thighs inward. Extend your tailbone to the floor and lift your pubis to the direction of the navel.

Keep the shoulder blades in the back, begin to spread them across and gently release them down your back. Lift the top part of the sternum in the direction of the ceiling while making sure that your ribs are not pushed forward. Spread your collarbones while you let your arms hang at each side of your torso.

Make sure that the crown of your head is balanced. The underside of your chin has to be parallel to the floor, your tongue is wide and flat to the mouth, and the throat and your gaze remain soft.

This kind of pose can be practiced in itself by keeping the position for up to a minute while you breathe easily. This is also the usual starting position of the standing poses.

2. Big Toe Pose (Padangusthasana)

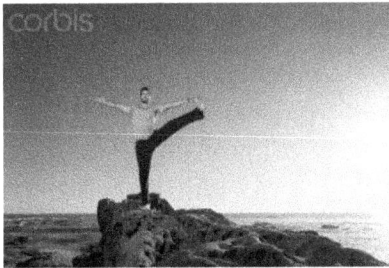

Stand straight with the inner part of your feet parallel and almost 6 inches apart from each other. Lift your kneecaps by contracting the front muscles of your thigh. Exhale while making sure that your legs remain straight and perform a forward bend from the hip joints, to your torso and head.

Slide the index and middle fingers of your two hands in the center of the big toes and the second toes. Curl your fingers under and get a firm grip with your big toes. Wrap the thumbs around the other two fingers in order to make the grip more secure.

You will then press the toes against the fingers. If in the beginning you are finding it hard to reach your toes without exerting too much effort on your back, you can pass straps beneath the balls of your feet and you will instead hold onto the straps.

As you inhale, you will lift your torso as if you are going to stand up and by extending your elbows. Stretch the front part of your torso, exhale and lift your sitting bones. As you perform the action, begin releasing your hamstrings and hollow the part below your navel in order to lift it slightly towards the back part of your pelvis.

While keeping your forehead relaxed, you will try to lift your sternum as high as you can. Make sure that you don't overdo the action to the point of compressing the back of your neck.

Inhale as you perform strong lifting of your torso while you continue to contract your front thighs. On the next exhalations, lift your sitting bones with force while you allow your hamstrings to relax. Make sure that you make the hollow in your lower back deeper.

Exhale and bend your elbows to the sides. Pull up on your toes and stretch the front and sides of your torso. Lower the torso in a gentle manner by doing a forward bend.

Hold the position for one minute. Lose the grip on your toes, put your hands to your hips and stretch your front torso. Inhale and swing your torso and head as if you are dealing with a single unit as you go back to an upright pose.

3. Chair Pose (Utkatasana)

knees, with your knees below the hips, the forearms on the floor and your shoulders placed above your wrists. Press your palms together in a firm manner.

Curl your toes, exhale and begin lifting your knees in a slightly bent manner and the heels lifted away from the floor. Extend your tailbone in the opposite direction of the back of your pelvis and then, you will press it in a slight manner in the direction of your pubis. As you feel the resistance at this point, begin lifting the sitting bones upward. Draw your inner legs up to your groins.

Keep your forearms pressed to the floor while your shoulder blades are firm against the back. Extend the blades and draw them in the direction of your tailbone. Keep your head between the upper arms and do not allow it to hang or get pressed against the floor.

It is okay to straighten your knees if the position is becoming uncomfortable. Keep extending your tailbone away from the pelvis and lift the upper part of the sternum away from the floor. Stay in this position for up to a minute. Release your knees as you exhale.

5. Downward-Facing Dog (Adho Mukha Svanasana)

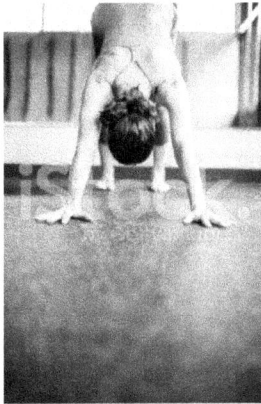

This is among the most popular yoga poses because it exercises the whole body and gives you a rejuvenating stretch. Begin with your hands and knees to the floor. Spread your palms, turn your toes under and keep your knees below your hips. Gently lift your knees as you exhale.

At first, keep the knees a little bent and the heels lifted. Extend your tailbone from behind your pelvis and press it in the direction of the pubis. As you feel the resistance, lift the sitting bones and draw your inner legs towards the groins.

Push the top parts of your thighs as you exhale and extend your heels to the floor. Straighten the knees without locking them. Make the muscles of the thighs firm as you roll the upper parts slightly inward. Make the front of the pelvis narrow.

Keep the bases of the index fingers pressed to the floor while the outer arms are firm. Lift the inner arms towards your upper shoulders while making sure that the shoulder blades remain firm behind the back. Extend your shoulder blades and begin drawing them into the tailbone, while your head remains between your upper arms.

6. Eagle Pose (Garudasana)

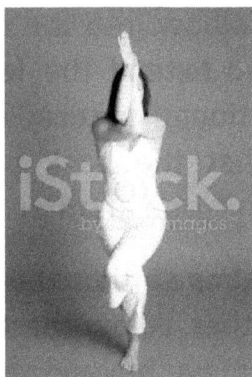

This pose is effective in giving you endurance, concentration, flexibility and strength. You will begin with the Tadasana pose. Slightly curve your knees and move your left foot in the direction of the ceiling. Keep the right foot balanced as the left thigh crosses over the other thigh. Position the left toes parallel to the floor, while you press the foot and hook the upper part of the foot at the back of your lower right calf. You need to keep your balance using your right foot.

Extend your arms, spreading the scapulas across the back part of the torso. Put the right arm at the top of the left, in front of your torso and begin bending your elbows.

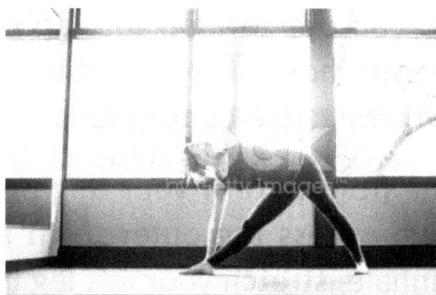

Begin in a Tadasana pose. As you exhale, step your feet up to four feet apart. Extend the arms parallel to the floor as you move each of them towards your sides with your palms facing down and your shoulder blades wide.

Slightly move your left foot to the right and the right foot out to the right on a 90-degree angle. Keep the right and left heels aligned. While keeping the thighs firm, turn the right thigh outward until the middle of the kneecap is aligned with the middle of the right ankle. Slightly roll your left hip forward, and then to the right as you rotate the upper part of the torso to the left.

Lift the inner part of the left groin deep into your pelvis in order to anchor the left heel to the floor. As you exhale, start bending the right knee over the right ankle. This will make your shin perpendicular to the floor.

Make your shoulder blades firm against the back of your ribs. Stretch your left arm upwards, turn the left palm in the direction of your head and inhale as you reach the arm towards the back of your left ear with your palm facing the floor. Extend your left heel as you lengthen the left side of your body. Make your head turn in the direction of your left arm, release the right shoulder away from the ear. Create equal length along both sides of your torso.

When you exhale, put the right side of your torso down to the top of your right thigh. Press your palm on the floor near the outer part of your right foot. Keep on pushing your right knee against the inner part of the arm, while you create a tension by putting your tailbone to the back of your pelvis to the direction of the pubis. The inner part of your right thigh at this

143

point has to be parallel to the long edge of your mat.

Hold the pose up to a minute. Inhale as you begin to come up. Push your heels to the floor with force and extend the left arm forcefully upwards. Reverse the position of your feet and repeat the sequence. Return to the Tadasana pose when you are done.

9. Extended Triangle Pose (Utthita Trikonasana)

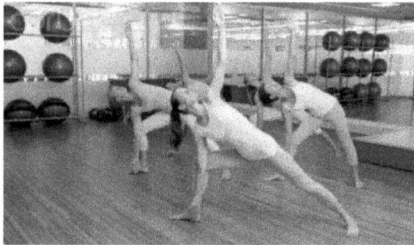

Begin in the Tadasana pose. Exhale and step until your feet are up to 4 feet apart. Extend your arms, keeping them parallel to the floor and actively reach to the sides with your palms down and the shoulder blades wide.

Turn the left foot in a slight manner to the right direction and the right foot out to the right at a 90-degree angle. Keep both heels aligned. Make the thighs firm as you turn the right thigh in an outward manner until the middle of the right kneecap is parallel to the middle of your right ankle.

Exhale and stretch your torso to the right as you bend from the hip joint. Strengthen the left leg as you perform the movement and press the outer part of the leg steadily to the floor. Perform a rotation of the torso to the left direction while the two sides remain equally long. Allow your hip to come forward in a slight manner as you extend the tailbone to the back heel.

Let your right hand rest on your shin or on the floor outside of the right foot. Extend your left arm upward while keeping it in line with the top parts of the shoulders. Your head should be in a neutral position

Chapter 17: More Benefits Of Yoga

On top of all of the benefits that I have already mentioned in this book, yoga provides even more. In this chapter, I want to go over all of the benefits that you can expect to see when you practice yoga on a regular basis. I want to make sure that you understand yoga must be practiced on a REGULAR basis in order for you to see these benefits. Yoga will not cure anything if you use it sporadically. If you want to see benefits, you will have to do it at least three times per week. As you become more advanced you can practice it more.

1.Yoga can help to decrease blood pressure by increasing circulation and oxygenation throughout the body.

2.A slower pulse indicates that you have a strong heart because it is able to pump more blood through it in fewer beats. When you practice yoga regularly, you will find that you have a lower pulse rate thus a stronger heart.

3.Yoga helps improve circulation of blood throughout the entire body because it helps to transport the nutrients that you eat as well as oxygen throughout the body. This means that you will have healthier organs, healthier skin, nails, hair and a healthier brain.

4.Many people suffer from respiratory issues and this is why they do not regularly exercise but yoga helps the lungs to work more efficiently. When you practice yoga regularly the rate at which you breathe, or your respiratory rate will slow down. This is because of the controlled breathing exercises that you are practicing while you are doing yoga poses as well as an increased fitness level.

5.Yoga also helps to massage the internal organs which helps them prevent diseases throughout the entire body. On top of this, you will become more attuned to your body and become more aware when something is not functioning the way that it should be functioning.

6.Yoga also helps to boost immunity, which means that you will get sick less often. When you do get sick, you will find that your symptoms are not as bad as they were before you began practicing yoga. Many people are suffering with autoimmune disorders today and it is caused much of the time by what the person eats. When you boost your immune system you will see less flare ups of the autoimmune disorders.

7.One of the great benefits of yoga is that in increases your pain tolerance. Many people who are suffering from chronic pain such as back pain find that after they begin practicing yoga, they no longer suffer from the pain.

8.Yoga helps to balance metabolism, which will result in a healthy weight and it will help you to control your hunger as well.

9.Yoga will help to stimulate detoxification in the body which has been shown to help delay the signs of aging.

10.One of the natural benefits of yoga is that you will have better posture. This is because while you practice yoga you are focusing not only on your breathing but your posture as well. When you become more aware of your posture, it is more likely to improve.

11.Many people think that yoga is for a person that is weak, but the fact is, since you are using your own body weight instead of training with conventional weights, you will build strength in each area of your body.

12.Regularly practicing yoga will increase the amount of energy that your body has each day. If you are practicing yoga correctly, you will have more energy after a session which is one reason that you should schedule your yoga sessions in the morning versus before you are getting ready for bed.

13.Because yoga benefits both the mind and the body, many people who practice yoga find that they sleep better at night

quality between the forced variety of concentration, and the voluntary sort of concentration.

Dharana can be described as the second example used. It is the immersive and voluntary surrender to the object on which you have placed all of your cognitive faculties. When you have had that experience, think back to the level of peace it provided and how refreshed you feel when you come out of it.

It is also one of the reasons there are large numbers of people who subconsciously search for problems to solve. Most minds focus when they are faced with problems to solve. They come out of that exercise feeling refreshed and light. That creates a reward. The mind then realizes that to feel that way again, it needs to solve another problem, so it goes in search of another problem, and then solves that. If it finds there are no problems to solve, the mind ends up making one. When the mind makes up a problem it is seen as self-sabotage.

Placing one's self in a dire predicament so that the mind can figure a way out is the classical western definition of self-sabotage. The solution is as easy as redirecting the powerful mind to areas of concentration and teach it to focus its faculties on more productive endeavors.

Dharana is a critical higher component of Yoga which is only approached once the other five have been attempted. One does not need to be an expert at the prior five limbs to be able to begin this one, but certain habits should have manifested by this point. For instance, breathing and effortless seating that one finds in Asana will be a good skill to have trained by this point.

One of the distractions that disturb the ability to concentrate is the numbing of different muscle groups or the strain in a particular muscle group that comes from either improper posture or poor breathing. When the muscle gets taxed and tired, or there is an acid build-up, it aches and pulls the mind away from what it is doing. As the practice to sit well develops, and one can perform a certain posture for a prolonged period, the mind is relieved of a possible source of distraction.

The same can be said for the need to eat. If one can control the habit of eating or the habit to do certain things at a certain time, all these will stop being distractions, and the mind will be able to concentrate on doing the thing that you have directed it to do.

The skill that was developed by pulling back all the sensations will also help in the concentration of the mind. As you realize that the various limbs of the Yoga, from the posture to the movement, to the reduction of stimuli that can distract, to the reduction of concerns, have all led to this point in the Yoga journey that allows the mind to focus on something and develop a thought. This concentration is important. It is not meditation, yet, but without concentration, there cannot be meditation,

It is common these days for folks to seek meditation and find solace in its promise of solutions. What most people miss is the need for the body to be able to get to a place where it can concentrate. Without it, all bets are off.

Enlightenment and peace can only be unearthed by the mind in a state of deep concentration. Without building on this ability the effort of Yoga will always only be merely a physical stretching exercise. It is often said that one needs to silence his or her mind. It is not the mind that needs to be silenced. It is the mind that needs to be directed and channeled to stop hearing the chatter. We are powerless to stop the chaos in the world around us, but we are fully capable of turning the sound off in our minds.

We are not capable of stopping the cogitations of the mind. It would be like asking the heart to stop beating. It exists because it does. However, the cognitive process that kicks up thoughts and triggers memories by association does not need to

157

thought. Concentrating on one thought will lead to the thoughts that are associated with it, and then the pond will be full of ripples again. Focus on your breath without priority. Our instinct to prioritize is where some of the inability to focus comes from. In this case, we never think of concentrating on breathing because it is never a priority. Imagine that it is. Right now, that is the only thing is important.

Once you can fix your mind on breathing, you will begin to see how easy it is and how refreshed you feel when you open your eyes and come out of it.

In time, you will expand this practice to other areas of your life. You will not need to seclude yourself in any sensory-deprived room. You will be able to direct your senses to the thing that you want to focus on. This is the ultimate goal. This is still not a state of meditation. It is merely concentration, and it is very powerful once you can do it at will.

CHAPTER 19: MEDITATION

Meditation is an important part of yoga. It deserves its own section, because it has such an important place in your yoga practice. While yoga often focuses a little more on the physical side with a secondary emphasis on mental health, meditation is more about mental health with a secondary emphasis on physical health. Even a few minutes of meditation each day can help you reduce stress levels significantly. And lowering your stress levels has the additional positive effect of reducing blood pressure, stabilizing heart and respiration rates, and boosting your immune system.

Meditation uses the standard stages of the mind to cause certain effects at certain times. Let's take a look at these different states.

Stage One: The Normal State of Mind

When your mind is in this state you are awake and being stimulated. You react normally, and you are thinking. During this phase your mind may jump around and wander a lot.You may be performing one task, and you may notice something that reminds you of something else and sends you off on a tangent. During this phase the mind is very active, but also very distractible. This can cause you a lot of problems if you're driving or working or doing something else that requires quite a lot of concentration.

This is the state of the mind in which stress tends to build up heavily. If your stress gets out of control you may find it very difficult to concentrate and you may start to fall behind on your work or daily tasks.

Stage Two: The Concentration State of Mind

During this phrase, you will enter the first state that carries you toward the state of meditation. Concentration isn't the state of meditation itself, but it is closer to it

are able to keep your thoughts centered onto one thing. You'll be able to concentrate on a particular thought and make it part of you.It will take you some time and practice to learn to control the stages of your mind, but you'll be rewarded with better concentration, better problem solving, and a great way to reduce stress.

Stage Four: The Contemplation State of Mind

The final level of meditation is the contemplation level. This is a very difficult level to understand without actually experiencing it for yourself. During this phase, you will enter a new type of consciousness. You've probably never entered this phase before, so it may be quite surprising the first time.Instead of focusing on your own issues as most people do, you will instead connect with the world itself. Your own body and mind will be completely secondary to you, and you will finally realize just how small we each are, and how very vast the universe is.It won't be easy to get to this phase. You may not reach it until you've practiced meditation many times. You were born with the ability to do this, but you have to actually practice it in order to achieve it.

The Purpose of Meditation

Meditation has many benefits. The most important one for many people is reaching enlightenment in the Contemplation phase, but this may not be important to everyone.Some people only want to use meditation as a way to become more spiritual, or do control stress or panic attacks, or to treat physical pain or illnesses. You don't have to meditate for the purpose of enlightenment or spirituality if that is of no interest to you. In fact, there are many people who don't even believe in spirituality of any kind but still use meditation as a way to relax and heal their mind and body.

Some executives use meditation as a way to ease their mind the way sleep does. In their busy lives, they may not get as much sleep as they really need, so they can use 5-10 minutes of meditation to refresh their mind when they feel stressed out, tired, distracted, or have trouble concentrating. Parents often use meditation as a way to calm the stress of daily life so they don't end up angry at their children. This is a great way to stay calm. Meditation is a very good anger management tool. If you have anger issues, you may use meditation as a way to get the condition under control.Let's look at some of the major benefits of meditation:

Meditation helps you focus more clearly. You'll be more efficient and you'll get more done in less time.Meditation will help you reduce your stress levels. Meditation will help you learn to be more sympathetic to other people, and more understanding. Mediation will help you become a kinder, more compassionate person. Meditation helps you communicate with others on a better, more effective level. Meditation can improve blood pressure, heart rate, and respiration, and even assist in managing heart disease. Meditation can help boost your immune system by lowering your stress levels. Meditation can help boost your memory and concentration through boosting oxygen levels. Meditation can help your mind achieve the kind of clarity you never thought you could experience. These are just a few of the different benefits you may achieve through meditation. There are so many additional benefits that are experienced by different people it would be very difficult to list them all here!

Types of Meditation

There are a lot of different types of meditation. You will discover that there are the ancient meditation methods that have been practiced for thousands of years, and there are also simpler modern methods that can be used. Ancient types of meditation are generally used to achieve enlightenment and each a high level of spirituality. If you plan to take the path to true enlightenment, you will probably want to learn one of those ancient methods. If you just want to use meditation to improve your physiological and/or psychological health, you can learn some of the simpler modern methods.

Concentrative Meditation

Concentrative meditation focuses on controlled breathing. In this method, you focus on your breathing while you also focus on a specific item, image, or sound.In this type of meditation, you may use mantras, or chants. This is the type of meditation you may have seen on television or in movies where people chant "O-mmmm". By concentrating on your breathing, you accomplish two important things. First, you learn to control your breathing. You can learn to adjust your respiration rate on the fly, which can really help you if you are prone to panic attacks.

Second, you learn to focus heavily. By concentrating on controlling your breathing, your mind is forced to focus on that one, rhythmic thing – your breathing. As you focus heavily on it, your mind will relax further and further into a meditative state. To practice this type of meditation, you will sit somewhere very quiet and comfortable and close your eyes. Focus carefully on the movement of their air in and out of your lungs. Think of nothing but your breathing. You may want to stare at a candle or hum or chant while you do this, especially if you have trouble concentrating. Sometimes the monotone sound or the gentle flicker of the candle can really help you concentrate as fully as you need to.

You will soon notice that your breathing will slow down and become much more regular than before. Your mind will start to ease, and you'll start to notice a feeling of calmness and serenity. This is one of the best methods for controlling stress, calming anger, and aiding focus in people who have memory or concentration issues.

Mindfulness Meditation

Mindfulness meditation is very different from concentrative. You won't focus on a single picture or sound, you'll instead focus on a broader picture. This one is a bit more difficult to perform, because it's a little harder to bring yourself to a meditative state while focusing on so much at once. It will be easy once you've practiced it for a while, but at first it may be quite difficult. As you sit in a quiet place, you'll take notice of the serene and beautiful things around you. Try to make this a place where you are happiest. Don't attempt this in any place that many evoke negative emotions.

You should be sitting as erect as possible so energy can flow through you as much as possible. Keep your back straight, and don't rotate your hips. Keep your head held high, but make sure your neck or back aren't so rigid that you become uncomfortable. Gaze downward, but don't close your eyes. Don't stare at any one single object, but instead let everything go out of focus. Your breath should be natural and relaxed, and you should strive to breathe as naturally as possible. Just let the breath flow in an out, relaxing you as it does.If your mind starts to wander to negative thoughts, simply think in your head that you are meditating right now and you will not allow these negative thoughts to interrupt your tranquility.

For as long as you feel comfortable, simply sit and absorb your surroundings. Listen to those pleasant sounds you hear around you, but try to block out any that may bother you. If you need help blocking out sounds, you can play nature CDs like waterfalls, thunderstorms, or beaches.

What Happens When You Meditate? During meditation, you will probably experience all or most of the following: Regulated breathing. Your breathing will become more regular and refreshing. Your heart and pulse rates will decrease. Your brain waves will change as you enter a relaxed state of mind. The production of the stress hormone cortisol will be decreased, which can help you get rid of belly fat. Your metabolic rate will decrease by about 20%, which may prolong your life. Your mind and body will enter a state of rest that may even be more important and restful than sleep. You may become more creative than ever before. Your blood pressure may fall a bit, especially if you normally have high blood pressure. Your muscles will relax and release their tension.

Oxygen will get to your muscles and brain more efficiently. You will be in a state somewhat like sleep or hypnosis, yet you will be fully alert. If you want to find out more about meditation, there are some excellent books on the subject. DVDs may also be very helpful, and there are a number of CDs that are designed to be used in meditation. Guided meditation CDs may be especially helpful in the beginning. They play special tones that eliminate your need to chant a mantra, and they also tell you step-by-step how to enter the correct state.

You may have to try a number of these CDs before you find one that works well for you. Although all or most of them will probably work, different people will respond in different ways to different voices, tones, sounds, and methods. Meditation should be a part of your yoga practice. It will help your mind and body in many ways, and you will experience more of the beneficial effects of yoga than you would without meditation.

contact with the floor. Sit on your heels and calm your body.

Now, move your butt toward the ground, so as to rest it on the floor. Once in position, your ankles should be in contact with the outer region of your hips. For proper practice, make sure you sit up very straight and do not bend, but be comfortable. If you feel excess stress or pressure on your hips or knees, you can continue in the Vajrasana position by sitting on your heels.

During the Sudarshan Kriya Yoga, breathe regularly and comfortably. A three part breath cycle is applied in Sudarshan Kriya, which requires practice.

In the first cycle, you need to breathe in and out normally with the equally spaced breaths. In the second cycle, your exhalations should double the time duration of the inhalation. In the third cycle, your inhalations should be twice the exhalation duration.

Advantages of practicing vajrasan in Sudarshan Kriya

The sitting posture Vajrasan is also known by several other names based on interpretation, physical nature or through the effect. It is known as Thunderbolt Pose, Pelvic Pose, Kneeling Pose, Adamantine Pose or Diamond Pose. The posture has a very significant role to play in effective yoga meditation, especially in Sudarshan Kriya Yoga. There are several benefits associated with vajrasan like:

-Mental stability

-Better concentration levels

-Cures digestive problems

-Natural back painkiller

-Cures stomach disorders

-Cures problematic conditions related to urine

-Amplifies blood circulation

-Minimize/Restrict obesity

-Tones the thigh muscles

-Acts as painkiller for arthritis patients

Inculcating OM chanting in Sudarshan Kriya

Chanting om is very effective and beneficial as it absorbs all the positive effect of Brahma, Vishnu and Shiva energy in the body. Brahma in Hindu mythology is the creator i.e. it betters our creativity skills like writing, drawing and other skills. Vishnu means one who continues and does not give up i.e. excellent management skills like volunteers, event coordinators. Shiva, the last principle, means destroyer i.e. dynamic professions like doctor, engineer, etc.

Accumulation of negative toxins has become a large part of our lives due to things like high-stress levels, anxiety, tension and many more that have become too common amongst us. This has led to people developing different diseases such as cardiovascular ailments, asthma, and cancer. Therefore, it is very important to have some peace of mind, which can be attained by practicing this yoga daily. It gives you immaculate mental abilities to deal with all problems while maintaining good health. It also betters your thinking capability, clarity of speech and feel harmonic and in accordance. Although it is not an easy technique, there have to be several trial counts to spread the energy to the companion chain for everyone. Regular Kriya practitioners have reported amplified immunity, increased stamina and sustained high-energy levels. It will also help you understand complex emotions like happiness, anger and sadness effectively.

Moreover, Sudarshan Kriya Yoga exercise does not have any particular side effects as it can be taught from both ends while keeping the effect on the body constant. This is becoming so popular and it is important that you start practicing too.

CHAPTER 21: YOGA MUDRAS PRACTICE FOR ANXIETY

Kalesvara Mudra.

This mudra allows you to shape and control the mind. It's primary benefit is to calm anxieties, but it is also known to heal addictions or unwanted character traits. It also enhances memory and concentration. As when practicing all mudras, it helps to set a positive intention at the onset or during the time practicing the mudra.

How to form the mudra: The pads of the middle fingers touch each other and extend, as do the pads of the thumbs. Curl the index, ring and pinky fingers in towards the palm of the hand and connect these fingers from the joint to the tips. Point the thumbs towards your chest with your elbows out to the side.

About Hasta Mudras

A hasta mudra is a gesture or positioning of the hands to channel and direct energy in the body. Mudras come from the over three thousand year old tradition of yoga originating in India. Hasta means "hand" in Sanskrit and "mudra" comes from the Sanskrit word "mud", meaning to delight. A mudra is a seal as in sealing your connection with the Divine or sealing energy in the body. There are many forms of mudras, such as with the eyes and the tongue.

Yoga is a spiritual practice and offers practical healing applications that benefit even those who aren't spiritually oriented. Hasta mudras work in a way that can be compared to acupuncture or reflexology. By activating parts of the hand, a hasta mudra opens up channels of energy and sends messages to the brain.

Try the kalesvara mudra above during your daily meditation today. If you are sensitive energetically, you may receive immediate results. But if the benefit doesn't come quickly, be patient and consistent in your practice. Keep in mind though that while hasta mudras can offer great healing, no mudra is a substitute for medication or medical attention.

Since hasta mudras work to change the energy in the body and spirit, it's best if you incorporate conscious breathing with your practice. Breathe full and free on the inhale and exhale the breath out completely. Find a rhythm with the breath. Try to make the inhale and exhale the same length.

It also helps to set a positive intention as you form a hasta mudra and concentrate on this intention during the practice

Mudras can be held for various lengths of time. You may find that today's mudra may only need to be held for 30 seconds until you feel refreshed or try holding the mudra throughout your meditation. There are no set rules. Let your intuition guide you. Have fun and explore!

Yoga Mudras Practice For Diabetes

Increased stress levels, sedentary lifestyle, lack of sleep, uncontrolled eating habits etc. are some of the factors whydiabetes has emerged as one of the common diseases in a scary way. And allopathy shows no hope for a cure.it is better to adopt natural ways to keep the side-effects of allopathic medicines to the minimum. Yoga, a traditional Indian exercise and with a history of 5,000 years is considered a holistic approach for healing and prevention. With certain yoga mudras or hand gestures, insulin levels in a diabetic person can be controlled.

There are a certain set of yoga mudras for diabetes control.

Before you start practicing these mudras, there are certain things which you need to keep in mind.

Consult with your physician in case you are suffering from any other ailment, including cardiovascular diseases or breathing troubles.

Please avoid practicing the mudras after a heavy meal. However, make sure that your body has sufficient glucose levels while you practice.

It is advisable to practice the mudras early in the morning, preferably before 8 am, for optimum results. However, you can practice these in the evening as well. If you are new to yoga, then make sure that you practice the mudras under the supervision of a qualified guru.

The 5 Yoga Mudras for Diabetes that every diabetic should know are:

1. Surya Mudra – Sun Mudra:

Surya' is a Sanskrit word that means 'Sun'. This mudra is known to increase the fire within the human body that in turn ensures a better metabolic rate. Diabetics, in general, have poor metabolic rates which results in increased sugar levels and weight gain. Regular practice of this mudra will help boost metabolic rates, thus ensuring loss of weight and lowering of

186

sugar levels As Surya mudra activates the fire element and generates strong heat in the body The mudra also helps easing indigestion and associated problems.

2. Pran Mudra:

Pran Mudra for Diabetes

Also Known as the Mudra of Life, it helps in improving the vital force of life and activates your Mooladhara Chakra or root chakra. Thus, it empowers you wholly within.   Performing this mudra improves the vital force of life, empowers a person from within and improves diabetic condition.   The mudra, when practiced without fail, helps in detoxifying your body. Practicing this mudra alongside Apan Mudra has been proven to offer relief to those suffering from diabetes. 3. Apan Mudra – Mudra of Digestion:

Apan Mudra for diabetes

The mudra, also called the mudra of purification, is one of the easiest yoga mudras. Apan mudra brings about a harmony as aids in striking a better balance between the elements within the human body. Thus, it ensures that the unwanted toxins are flushed out properly from your body. Because of frequent urination it helps in eliminating the wastes, thus lowering the blood sugar levels.

4. Gyan Mudra – Mudra of Knowledge:

Gyan Mudra for diabetes

Also known as Chin Mudra, it can be practiced by the diabetics to enjoy deep relaxation. It helps in relaxing the body and eliminating stress and other mind-related issues.

5. Linga Mudra:

Linga Mudra for diabetes

Lingam, in Sanskrit, means phallus – the male reproductive organ. In Linga Mudra, the fire element in the body is activated which creates lot of heat. This leads to an increase in metabolic rate, loss of body weight and decrease of insulin levels.This, in turn, causes an increase in metabolic levels. The higher the metabolic levels, the more the chances of a person losing weight. This, automatically, lowers blood sugar levels, offering relief from diabetes.

Yoga Mudras Practice For Back Pain

As the name suggest, back mudra is effective in relieving back pain. Mudras are hand gestures that has healing properties. There is a specific mudra known as back mudra. This mudra is helpful in relieving back ache. Mudra works in way which helps in balancing the energies in the body,hence helps to get rid of complications due to pain. back mudra is effective in relieving back pain. Hastapadasna is also good for back pain

Position in Back Mudra

There are separate mudras for right and left hands which has to be done in conjunction with each anothers.

Right hand:

1) Let thumb, middle and little fingers should touch at the tip

2) Extend the ring and index fingers.

Back Mudra - right hand gesture

Left hand:

1) Place your thumb joint on the nail of the index finger.

2) Extend the other fingers

Back Mudra is effective in relieving back pain

How long to practice back mudra to relieve back ache?

Do back mudra for four times a day for 4 minutes each. Or do it as long as it has effect on the acute back complaints.

Specialty of Back mudra

1) This mudra is very effective when someone with a weak back get engaged in an activity that strains the back too much

and causes painful tensions, such as gardening or cleaning work.

2) When someone has to sit for too long in the wrong position.

There are numerous causes that can cause Backaches. Too little sleep or rest or too little exercise can cause backache. Fears, heavy meals, mental stress are other causes which can cause back ache. Some time toxins get deposited along the waste line, but that does not necessarily cause backache. So exercise is very important to get rid away waste accumulated. You can also read about some of the yoga asnas that helps body to get in shape.

Mudra meditation for reliving back ache

This mudra can be even more effective when done with mudra meditation.

• Keep your arms and spine straight and erect.

• Hold Fingers in the back mudra as explained above.

• Rest your hands on thighs or on table or chair or anything else, just to provide them a base. Or you can Keep the arms open to the sky. It is a pose for visualization of receiving cosmic energy. You can even lie down in open sky for this meditation.

• Inhale less than exhale. You can even lie down in open sky for this meditation.

• Focus on the part of the body where you have pain and visualise that it is released as you exhales.

Method of Back Pain Relieving Mudra

The thumb, middle finger and little finger of your right hand should gently touch one another, while the index and ring finger are extended.

Now place the thumb of your left thumb joint on the nail of the left index finger.

Perform this asana for four times in a day, for four minutes each.

You can even perform Mudra meditation for relieving your back pain. The following is its method:

Keep your arms and spine erect. Fingers in the mudra as explained above.

Rest your hands on thighs, table, chair handles, or on bed.

Keep the arms open to the sky (preferably). It is a visualisation of receiving cosmic energy.

You should be inhaling less than exhaling. You can even lie down in open sky for this meditation.

Focus on the pain and visualise that it is dissipating with each of your exhales.

Do not expect immediate results although that does happen from time to time. If it does not work out right away for you, do not be discouraged. This is the most holistic and comprehensive way of treating your back pain as well as having a permanently healthy back that you could have taken. Show yourself the same compassion that you would to someone else who suffered from pain. You can add a few more Yoga poses to your routine such as the Child's pose. Consult a good Yoga trainer for this.

CONCLUSION

I think it is vital for you to really take your yoga experience seriously and at a pace that suits you. Everyone is different and will feel differently about learning yoga. Some will find it difficult because they don't have the experience of switching off thought and feel that they cannot manage it. However, if you feel like this, use exercises which help to train the mind to switch off. One of the best is learning to relax and to do this is simple. Simply lie on the bed in a room with the curtains closed. Close your eyes and think of one part of your body, preferably your toes to start off with working through the different body parts right up to the top of the head. As you think of that body part, flex it and feel it move and then relax it.

During the relaxation exercises, you learn to think of nothing except the body parts and concentrate on the way that you are breathing. In through the nose, hold the breath for a moment and then out through the nose, making sure that the upper diaphragm is pivoting while you breathe. If you can't do this properly, place your hand on your chest/breast and as you breath out press down on your chest/breast area so that your body does that pivot action.

If you are intent on taking lessons, make sure that the instructor that you have is someone that you can work with. It's a good idea to visit a class and see what goes on because this gives you a great feeling for how well in tune the teacher is with the students. If you find that there is discomfort between them, you can try another teacher until you find one that you believe is right for you. You can't get on with everyone in this world but when you want to find a yoga teacher, remember you are entering a very spiritual practice and you need someone who is in tune with you and who you can really feel good about working with.

For further information on yoga moves, use YouTube but watch out for the qualifications of people who give demonstrations. There are some extremely useful teachers, and you may also like to download an app for your iPad or for your phone so that you can follow the movements given by instructors from there. The thing with modern technology is that it provides you with backup services in video format that is great when you are learning different positions.

This book has been written for the uninitiated and it is hoped that this journey that we have taken together has given you the basics, so that your yoga experience can really begin and you can start to feel the benefit of your yoga practice. Remember, you can lose weight. Remember that you can feel more complete in your life, but also remember that care of your body doesn't stop when you finish your session for the day. As stated in this book, your lifestyle will to a certain extent determine your success at losing weight and at achieving that spirituality and peace of mind that you seek. There is no quick cure for being overweight and there is no quick way to change the way that you think. This philosophy can and has changed millions of lives worldwide. Why? Because its roots are well planted and yoga has been proven to be a benefit to all who practice it on a regular basis.

Expect to feel differently about your life. Expect to feel a sense of wellbeing once you practice yoga on a regular basis. Expect yourself to become more sensible and sensitive to your body's needs. With the kind of care that goes hand in hand with yoga, your lifestyle will become fulfilling and as you achieve each exercise perfectly for the first time, you feel a sense of thrill at the achievement. These are not hard exercises to do, but watching yourself in a mirror can help you a lot when performing the exercises alone. You will be able to see the straightness of your back. You will be able to see how well formed the inverted V is when you do the poses. Getting the position right is more important than performing one particular exercise for so many times. Make sure that you look at what you are doing and that you set a limit for your daily exercise routine that doesn't push your body too hard too fast.

In conjunction with yoga, you can include walking as a wonderful exercise to compliment your yoga practice, since this takes you out into the fresh air and keeps you in tune with the world around you. Sitting in a park may bring on the feeling that you want to meditate. With practice you will be able to. Sitting by the sea, you may get that urge to do a sun salutation and that's possible too, but be sure to take your mat with you and to be suitably attired. When you embrace yoga and let it embrace your body, your life changes beyond measure and you start to see that it holds a lot more possibility than you thought. Your chakras are clear, the energy can flow in and out of your body easily and you will find that you are ill less frequently. It's all part and parcel of embracing this philosophy and getting nearer to your inner you. When your mind and body are in tune, this automatically means that you are able to find peace of mind and will have the ability to take strength from this liaison. Then, you will understand why people use yoga and what it is that strengthens your inner resolve to succeed.